Nephropathy: Beyond the Basics

Nephropathy: Beyond the Basics

Editor: Woody Bones

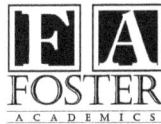

FA
FOSTER
A C A D E M I C S
www.fosteracademics.com

www.fosteracademics.com

FA
FOSTER
ACADEMICS

Cataloging-in-Publication Data

Nephropathy : beyond the basics / edited by Woody Bones.
      p. cm.
Includes bibliographical references and index.
ISBN 978-1-63242-707-6
1. Kidneys--Diseases. 2. Nephrology. I. Bones, Woody.
RC902 .N47 2019
616.61--dc23

Foster Academics,
118-35 Queens Blvd., Suite 400,
Forest Hills, NY 11375, USA

ISBN 978-1-63242-707-6 (Hardback)

Contents

Preface

This book aims to highlight the current researches and provides a platform to further the scope of innovations in this area. This book is a product of the combined efforts of many researchers and scientists, after going through thorough studies and analysis from different parts of the world. The objective of this book is to provide the readers with the latest information of the field.

Nephropathy refers to the disease of a kidney, which leads to kidney damage and loss of kidney function. The progression of nephropathy can vary from mild to serious, and can potentially result in kidney failure. This is end-stage kidney disease, which can be treated through a dialysis or a kidney transplant. Nephrosis and nephritis are kidney diseases that give rise to nephrotic and nephritic syndrome respectively. Chronic kidney disease leads to a gradual loss of kidney function over time, while in acute kidney disease, kidney function reduces within seven days. Kidney disease is caused due to a deposition of immunoglobulin A antibodies in the glomerulus, toxic effects of chemotherapeutic agents, analgesic administration, long-term exposure to lead, etc. A high risk of nephropathy is associated with chronic conditions such as diabetes mellitus, systemic lupus erythematosus and high blood pressure. The standard line of diagnosis involves review of medical history, physical examination, urine test and ultrasound of the kidneys. This book includes some of the vital pieces of work being conducted across the world, on various topics related to nephropathy. It strives to provide a fair idea about this clinical condition and to help develop a better understanding of the latest advances in the diagnosis and management of nephropathy. A number of latest researches have been included to keep the readers up-to-date with the global concepts in this area of study.

I would like to express my sincere thanks to the authors for their dedicated efforts in the completion of this book. I acknowledge the efforts of the publisher for providing constant support. Lastly, I would like to thank my family for their support in all academic endeavors.

Editor

Acute Kidney Injury (AKI)

Keiko Hosohata, Ayaka Inada, Saki Oyama and
Kazunori Iwanaga

Abstract

Acute kidney injury (AKI) is a serious public health issue, with an increasing incidence and significant associated deleterious effects. Several studies have reported the consequences of AKI, including prolonged hospital stay, increased healthcare costs, morbidity, and mortality. Many factors are known to affect AKI development. Kidney is exposed to a larger proportion and a higher concentration of drugs and toxins than other organs through the secretion of ionic drugs by tubular organic ion transporters across the luminal membranes of renal tubular epithelial cells and through reabsorption of filtered toxins into the lumen of the tubule; these cells are at a greater risk for injury. This section gives an overview of AKI including the definition, causes, and prognosis.

Keywords: acute kidney injury, drug, prognosis

1. Introduction

1.1. AKI definition

Acute kidney injury (AKI) results in an acute and usually transient decrease in renal function. AKI is defined as any of the following (not graded): (1) an increase in serum creatinine (SCr) by ≥ 0.3 mg/dl (≥ 26.5 mol/l) within 48 h, or (2) an increase in SCr to ≥ 1.5 times baseline that is known or presumed to have occurred within the prior 7 days, or (3) urine volume < 0.5 ml/kg/h for 6 h.

1.2. Clinical stratification of AKI

The RIFLE (Risk of renal dysfunction, Injury to the kidney, Failure of kidney function, Loss of kidney function and End-stage kidney disease) classification was proposed as a diagnostic criterion of acute renal failure (ARF) in order to ameliorate the morbidity and mortality of ARF (**Table 1**) [1–3]. Under this proposal, AKI has instead been proposed to be called ARF. In addition, the AKI Network (AKIN) was formed around the attendees of a critical care and kidney-related conference; the revised version of the RIFLE classification by the AKIN was proposed as the diagnostic criterion of AKI (**Table 2**) [4] and the Kidney Disease Improving Global Outcomes (KDIGO) were used for the diagnosis of AKI, where the clinical conditions are elevated serum creatinine level and a decreased urine output within 48 h (**Table 3**) [5].

SCr, serum creatinine; ESKD, end-stage kidney disease.

An abrupt (within 48 h) reduction in kidney function is currently defined as an absolute increase in serum creatinine of more than or equal to 0.3 mg/dl ($\geq$26.4 μmol/l), a percentage increase in serum creatinine of more than or equal to 50% (1.5-fold from baseline), or a reduction in urine output (documented oliguria of less than 0.5 ml/kg per hour for more than 6 h). AKI is diagnosed if one of the definitions in 1–3 is met. If a diagnosis is made based solely on urine output, this diagnostic criterion is used under the condition that body fluid volume is properly corrected and urinary tract obstruction or readily reversible oliguria are excluded. SCr, serum creatinine.

	Glomerular filtration rate (GFR)	**Urine output**
Risk	SCr more than 1.5 times or GFR decrease >25%	Less than 0.5 ml/kg/h for more than 6 h
Injury	SCr more than 2.0 times or GFR decrease >50%	Less than 0.5 ml/kg/h for more than 12 h
Failure	SCr more than 3.0 times, or GFR decrease >75%, or SCr $\geq$0.5 mg/dl with acute elevation SCr $\geq$4 mg/dl	Less than 0.3 ml/kg/h for more than 24 h or anuria for more than 12 h
Loss	Continued ARF (complete loss of kidney function) for more than 4 weeks	Continued ARF (complete loss of kidney function) for more than 4 weeks
ESKD	End-stage kidney disease (dialysis dependency for more than 3 months)	End-stage kidney disease (dialysis dependency for more than 3 months)

Table 1. RIFLE classification.

Stage	**SCr**	**Urine output**
Stage 1	Increase in SCr of more than or equal to 0.3 mg/dl or increase to more than or equal to 150–200% (1.5- to 2-fold) from baseline	Less than 0.5 ml/kg/h for more than 6 h
Stage 2	Increase in SCr to more than 200–300% (>2- to 3-fold) from baseline	Less than 0.5 ml/kg/h for more than 12 h
Stage 3	Increase in SCr to more than 300% (>3-fold) from baseline or SCr of more than or equal to 4.0 mg/dl with an acute increase of at least 0.5 mg/dl	Less than 0.3 ml/kg/h for 24 h or anuria for 12 h

Table 2. AKIN classification.

Stage	Classification standard by SCr	Classification standard by urine output
1	SCr more than 27 μmol/l (0.3 mg/dl) or SCr elevated to 1.5–1.9 times normal values	Less than 0.5 ml/kg/h within 6–12 h
2	SCr 2–2.9 times normal values	Less than 0.5 ml/kg/h in more than 12 h
3	SCr elevation to ≥3 times normal values or SCr ≥ 354 μmol/l (4.0 mg/dl) or start of renal replacement therapy	Anuria for 12 h

Table 3. KDIGO classification.

1.3. Classification of AKI

AKI is classified roughly into prerenal, renal, and postrenal according to the site of onset [6]. Prerenal refers to cases of a decreased blood flow to the kidney as a result of systemic illness. Renal refers to cases with roots in the kidney. Postrenal refers to cases caused by issues in the lower urinary tract (urinary duct, bladder, or urethral tube).

2. Drug-induced AKI

2.1. Definition

Drug-induced kidney injury (DKI) is a general term for newly occurring kidney injury or kidney injury that has been exacerbated by the drugs administered for diagnosis and treatment. Furthermore, DKI can be classified as follows: toxic kidney injury, acute interstitial nephritis by allergy mechanism (hypersensitivity kidney injury), drug-induced indirect toxicity through electrolyte abnormality and blood flow decrease, drug-induced crystal formation, and urinary tract obstruction kidney injury for calculus formation.

2.2. Etiology

Because primary urine, largely filtered by the glomeruli, is reabsorbed in the proximal tubules, drugs and metabolites are easily accumulated in high concentrations in the kidney. For this reason, the kidney is susceptible to drug-induced injury. Because primary urine becomes concentrated in the proximal tubules after primary urine is filtered from the glomeruli, tubular necrosis through direct toxicity occurs with an increased frequency in a dose-related fashion. Drug-induced kidney injury is defined by a new-onset disorder of the kidney or a further exacerbation of the existing dysfunction of the kidney by the administration of drugs. Furthermore, when patients have risk factors, such as older age (elderly), compromised renal function (chronic kidney failure), dehydration, frequent administration of drugs, and baseline disease (diabetes mellitus or myeloma), disorder of the kidney tends to take place. Drugs prone to cause disorder of the kidney may include nonsteroidal anti-inflammatory drugs (NSAIDs), antibiotics (aminoglycosides, new quinolones), immunomodulatory agents, contrasts (iodinated contrast), anticancer drugs (cisplatin), vitamin D and calcium preparations, and drugs for high blood pressure (RAAS blockade in particular) (**Table 4**).

2.3. Pathophysiological

The pathogenic mechanism of drug-induced AKI is poorly understood, but the following are known: the shift of hemodynamic status, the induction of acute interstitial nephritis, the induction of acute renal tubular injury, drug-induced thrombotic microangiopathy, the induction of glomerular nephritis, the induction by crystals in the tubular lumen, and others.

2.4. Kidney hemodynamic change

GFR, which is determined by glomerular pressure and filtration coefficients, is reduced by the inability to maintain glomerular pressure due to renal hemodynamic alterations, which are dependent on the renin-angiotensin aldosterone system (RAAS), endothelin system, prostaglandin system, and nitric oxide (NO). In addition, this condition occurs with minimal change in the vascular smooth muscle of the afferent renal arteriole and the efferent renal arteriole. Non-steroidal anti-inflammatory drugs (NSAIDs) are well-known offending agents and are associated with a high proportion of cases. Compared with internal medications, topical medicines have not been seen as a problem; however, recently, anti-inflammatory

Classification	Prospective drug
Renal hemodynamic alteration	NSAIDs, renin-angiotensin system drugs, active vitamin D, calcineurin inhibitors (ciclosporin and tacrolimus), and diuretics
Thrombotic microangiopathy (TMA)	Angiogenesis inhibitors (VEGF inhibitors), gemcitabine, mitomycin C, interferon, mTOR inhibitors, thienopyridine (antiplatelet drugs), kinin, oxymorphone (opioid), oral contraceptives, and calcineurin inhibitors
Acute renal tubular injury	General chemotherapy (cisplatin, ifosfamide, etc.), antibacterial drugs (aminoglycosides, amphotericin B, vancomycin, etc.), zoledronic acid, BRAF inhibitors, ALK inhibitors, iron chelators, heavy metals, and contrasts
Acute tubulointerstitial nephritis (AIN)	NSAIDs, antibacterial drugs (β-lactam, sulfa drugs, quinolones), diuretics, and PPI
Intratubular obstruction (crystalluria)	Crystal deposition-induced renal disease: antiviral drugs (cisplatin, ifosfamide, etc.), antibacterial drugs (sulfa drugs, ciprofloxacin), methotrexate, triamterene, ascorbic acid, sodium phosphate (laxative), warfarin
Glomerulonephritis	Membranous nephropathy: NSAIDs, platinating agents, bucillamine, and penicillamine
	MCD: NSAIDs, lithium, interferon, pamidronate, vaccines
	FSGS: in addition to the above, hormonal agents and heroin
	lupus nephritis: methyldopa, hydralazine, procainamide, and quinidine
Others	liquorice root, vitamin D, and antithrombotic agents (Warfarin)

MCD, minimal change disease; FSGS, focal segmental glomerular sclerosis.

Table 4. Causes of drug-induced AKI.

analgesic plasters containing NSAIDs that achieve comparatively higher blood levels have been sold; these forms of administration should also be considered. NSAIDs decrease blood flow in the afferent renal arteriole and GFR by blocking the production of prostaglandins. COX-2-selective inhibitors have turned out to be a cause of AKI development as well as COX-2-nonselective inhibitors, so attention should be paid to these inhibitors regardless of their mechanisms. In addition, RASS inhibitors cause the efferent renal arteriole to dilate and decrease GFR. These drugs have a protective effect for the kidney in CKD patients in the mid- and long term; however, our attention to AKI is required under circumstances where it is easy to reduce renal blood flow.

2.5. Causes of drug-induced thrombotic microangiopathy (drug-induced TMA)

TMA describes a disorder that is thought to be an aftereffect of pathological microvascular endothelial damage and has the three following features: hemolytic anemia, thrombocytopenia, and organ damage. Drugs may induce TMA in some instances, especially angiogenesis inhibitors such as vascular endothelial growth factor (VEGF) and anticancer drugs such as bevacizumab, which carry greater risks. It is thought that VEGF produced by glomerular podocytes is needed to maintain the function of endothelial cells and epidermal cells [7]. A high blood pressure and albuminuria are more problematic in drug-induced TMA; conversely, hemolytic anemia is less problematic. Aside from VEGF inhibitors, it is known that interferon and calcineurin inhibitors could increase drug-induced TMA that shows evidence of thrombocytopenia and schistocytes and signs in glomerular endothelial cells.

2.6. Causes of tubular damage

Drugs taken up by renal tubular epithelial cells mainly cause necrosis in the proximal tubule and apoptosis in the distal tubule and then cast formation in the tubular lumen and blockage by cells that fall behind into the renal tubule lumen, which consequently deteriorate quickly. The following drugs produce renal tubular injury and acute tubular necrosis (ATN) as symptoms progress: antineoplastic drugs such as cisplatin and ifosfamide, antibacterial drugs such as aminoglycosides, and antifungals such as amphotericin B. As a result of renal tubular injury, nephrogenic diabetes insipidus (NDI) and Fanconi syndrome are present. In the case of vancomycin, the pathogenesis of kidney injury is thought to occur as a result of increasing oxidant stress [8] in the proximal kidney tubule, with casts appearing in the kidney tubule [9]. As risk factors, nephrotoxic drugs (aminoglycosides), in combination with high-dose diuretics (4 g/day) and a high level of trough (≥20 µg/ml), patients in ICU for more than 1 week of treatment period is known. In addition, calcineurin inhibitors are recommended for therapeutic drug monitoring (TDM) for concentration-dependent development in the proximal kidney tubule.

2.7. Causes of acute interstitial nephritis

AIN involves drug-induced delayed hypersensitive reactions such as fever, rash, articular inflammation, or hepatic disorder in combination with declining kidney function, mainly involving neutrophil, T lymphocyte, and monocyte invasion in the renal stroma. However, these extrarenal manifestations are not inevitable and furthermore present with symptoms of nephrosis with tiny variation at times. Drug-induced AIN occurs with a high frequency. Often, kidney injury occurs a few days to a few weeks after administration of the offending drug, especially antibacterial drugs, such as beta-lactam agents, quinolone agents, and rifampicin, which are all causes of AIN; however, the cases caused by NSAIDs and proton pump inhibitors (PPIs) have tended to increase. Immune checkpoint inhibitors (e.g., PD-1 inhibitor), such as nivolumab, which recently has rapidly been expanded to apply to numerous bacterial species, have been reported to increase kidney injury, including interstitial nephritis.

2.8. Tubule occlusion by crystals (crystal nephropathy)

The drug concentration in the renal tubule lumen increases in order to acidify urine by urinary concentration and excretion of H in the distal convoluted tubule. Under these acidic conditions, crystallization of the drug occurs, inducing a nephropathy called crystal nephropathy. Antiviral drugs such as acyclovir and indinavir and methotrexate are known to cause kidney disorders due to drug-related crystal deposition in the renal tubules. There are many cases where casts are lost into the urine. Psychotropic agents and rhabdomyolysis-inducing drugs, such as statin medications or fibrates, are included in this category because obstruction of the renal tubule by myoglobin is possible. Excessive use of common supplements such as vitamin C carries a danger of promoting oxalic acid crystals.

2.9. Causes of glomerulonephritis-related damage

Glomerulonephritis induces functional disorder by blocking resorption in the renal tubule. The relation between rheumatoid arthritis agents, such as platinating agents or bucillamine and membranous nephropathy and antihypertensive drugs, such as methyldopa or hydralazine and drug-induced lupus kidney inflammation, has been highlighted for some time. Interferon used in clinical application for the treatment of hepatitis, however, has been reported to induce minimal change disease (MCD) or focal segmental glomerular sclerosis (FSGS) [10]. In addition, a relationship between NSAIDs and membranous nephropathy or MCD has been indicated.

2.10. Contrast-induced nephropathy (CIN)

CIN is diagnosed in the case of kidney function declines after the administration of contrast in the absence of other causes (e.g., cholesterol embolus). The mechanism of CIN remains to be completely elucidated; however, the following factors have been considered: (1) a decrease in oxygen supply due to blood vessel spasm in the renal medulla, causing direct toxicity to the renal tubule, (2) a decreased renal perfusion by increased adenosine and endothelin or reduced carbon monoxide [11]; coexisting risk factors such as kidney function disorder, advanced age (more than 75 years old), dehydration, cardiac failure, agents (diuretic agents, NSAIDs, aminoglycoside antibiotics, and vancomycin), diabetes mellitus, and multiple myeloma; in particular, kidney function disorder is the greatest risk factor. In addition, diabetes mellitus, which has become recognized as a risk factor, is considered a factor in itself and promotes a further elevated risk for the development of CIN in CKD patients through its complications. Gadolinium (Gd) contrast agents, including extracellular liquid Gd contrast agents and hepatocyte-specific Gd contrast agents, are classified as linear and macrocyclic or as ionic and nonionic on the basis of their chelate structure. Gd is a heavy metal element and is highly poisonous in the case of direct administration. Therefore, Gd is administered as a chelate so that it is excreted into the urinary tract (and partly into the biliary tract) without metabolizing inside the body. Adverse events of Gd contrast agents occur in three types: acute adverse effect, occurring within 1 h after intravenous injection; delayed adverse effect, occurring from 1 h to 1 week after intravenous injection; and super-delayed adverse effect, such as nephrogenic systemic fibrosis (NSF), which occurs more than 1 week or even several years after intravenous injection. Moreover, there is a newly recognized problem that Gd remains in the brain without causing kidney disorder [12]. Many subsequent studies have reported that residual Gd in the body is more linear type than macrocyclic type [13, 14] and remains not only in the brain but also throughout the whole body when the residual volume is increased in the presence of kidney disorder [15]. Complications caused by residual Gd have not been reported; however, patients who are frequently exposed to contrast generally have some kind of chronic disease, so the effects of residual Gd may be obscured or misinterpreted as subjective or objective evidence of their disease. Notably, in the case of Gd remaining in the brain, Gd deposits in neuronal nuclei have been observed by electronic microscopy [16]. Gd is not liberated very well; its thermodynamic stability constant and condition stability constant are high, leading to a high chelate stability. Its half-life at pH = 1.0 represents the time required to liberate half of Gd from the chelate under pH = 1.0, but it remains stable much longer under other conditions. In general, linear type chelates have a lower stability than macrocyclic chelates [17].

2.11. Other etiologies

There are cases that result from electrolyte abnormalities; for example, the abnormal use of diuretic drugs or glycyrrhiza causes kidney disorder by hypokalemia and excess administration of vitamin D preparation causes kidney disorder via hypercalcemia. In addition, warfarin, which has been in use as an anticlotting drug for many years, has been reported to easily cause kidney disorders, particularly when PT-INR exceeds 3; however, the mechanism has yet to be determined [18]. Among the pathological findings of kidney disorder due to warfarin, red blood cell casts have been observed with high frequency.

2.12. Clinical presentation of drug-induced AKI

Symptoms appear within a few hours or a few years after taking or using the offending agents, and in some cases, no symptoms appear. Renal tubular injury sometimes presents with the following symptoms: polyuria, urinary frequency, thirst, fatigue, and anorexia. Skin rash, joint pain, fever, and hematuria are observed as signs of allergy. In the case of thrombotic microangiopathy, purple spots and bleeding tendency with thrombopenia appear in the soft palate and the extremities. In the presence of crystal nephropathy, knock pain is commonly observed dorsally and bilaterally with postrenal acute renal failure. With progression, acute or chronic renal failure develops.

2.13. Diagnosis of drug-induced AKI

The size of the kidney is normal or swollen. The elevation of urinary N-acetyl-β-glucosaminidase (NAG) or L-type fatty acid binding protein (L-FABP) is observed with a urine test. In particular, the proteinuria is of low grade (less than 1 g/day) and associated with renal tubule dysfunction (mainly β_2-microglobulin). However, the urinary findings depend on the presence or absence of glomerular lesions. The detection of urinary eosinophils has been used for the diagnosis of drug-induced AKI [19], but is weak evidence for clinical judgment, as it has a lower positive-predictive rate and a higher false-negative rate than other markers. Renal hemodynamic type is rarely examined, but hyperkalemia is presented in patients receiving drugs related to the RAA system. Thrombotic microangiopathy is commonly associated with thrombocytopenia, an appearance of schistocytes, and elevation of lactate dehydrogenase (LDH). In acute tubular necrosis, muddy brown casts are observed in the urinary sediment. The examination of accumulation enhancement in the kidney by gallium scintigraphy is used for the diagnosis of acute interstitial nephritis related to antibacterial drug overdose, but this is not a common diagnostic approach because it is difficult to distinguish between drug accumulation and infection or glomerular disease. Then, there is the problem of the low specificity of the drug-induced lymphocyte stimulation test (DLST), which is used to examine the patient's blood in cases of suspected drug-related AKI. In crystal nephropathies, urinary crystals or high-brightness echo on renal ultrasonography due to crystals may be observed. Renal biopsy is not essential for diagnosing drug-induced AKI, and it is considered to produce a hangover of kidney disorder after drug withdrawal or maintain uric protein in the nephrotic range and glomerular hematuria.

2.14. Treatment of drug-induced AKI

The treatment is essentially discontinuing use of the suspected drugs; treatment also includes proper maintenance of body fluid volume and blood pressure, and sometimes, the use of rehydration or diuretics to maintain adequate perfusion of the kidney. We consider using kidney replacement therapy in cases where the following symptoms are observed: a marked elevation of BUN or hyperkalemia, pulmonary edema that fails to respond to diuretics, or uremic symptoms. In the treatment of drug-induced acute interstitial nephritis, we may consider steroid therapy after early withdrawal of drugs (within 2 weeks), when kidney disorder hangover occurs under the discontinuation of the suspected drug [20]. We use upward of 1 mg/kg/day steroid for a short period, but there are no large-scale studies related to patient characteristics or symptoms that indicate this therapy. In addition, alkalinization of the urine with baking soda or acetazolamide treatment is used to promote the solubility of crystals in the case of kidney disorder caused by the deposition of methotrexate crystals in the renal tubules. Methotrexate has a low molecular weight of 454.44, its protein binding rate is 50%, and it is removed rapidly from plasma; because of these factors, a combination of plasma exchange and hemodialysis with a high-flux membrane is effective. A recombinant enzyme preparation that directly decomposes methotrexate has already been developed in Europe and the United States. Contrast nephropathy rarely needs specific treatment to resolve. With a lower residual renal function or oliguria, treatment is needed for advanced CKD. It is said that the aggressive introduction of blood purification therapy as well as other AKI avoidance is helpful to reduce case fatality rate and complications such as progression of kidney disorder. Treatments such as diuretics, human atrial natriuretic peptide, and low-dose dopamine have been considered by now, but these treatments are not recommended, as their usefulness has not yet been demonstrated. Thus, it is necessary to consider fluid therapy after CIN and important to carefully select the infusion volume after evaluating body fluid volume because an excessive increase in fluid could elevate the case fatality rate.

3. Nondrug-induced AKI

3.1. Heart function and AKI

There are many important factors related to both the heart and the kidney that indicate the following pathway leading to kidney disorder or cardiac arrest (**Figure 1**) [21]. Patients who have suffered acute decompensated heart failure tend to develop AKI during the course of treatment, which is known to worsen renal function despite the correction of heart function [22, 23]. Kidney function disorder results in heart function disorder, and this connection has recently been referred to as cardiorenal syndrome (CRS). Ronco et al. classified clinical conditions into five groups, divided by acute and chronic [24]. In this classification, we give an outline of types CRS1 and CRS3, related to heart function and AKI.

3.2. Hepatorenal syndrome

3.2.1. Pathogenesis of hepatorenal syndrome

The arterial vasodilation theory is universally recognized as underlying hepatorenal syndrome [25]. With progression, hepatic cirrhosis and vascular resistance are reduced, and blood pressure is decreased by vasodepressor factors such as carbon monoxide and cannabinoids [26]. At the early stage of hepatic cirrhosis, compensatory mechanisms such as the elevation of cardiac pumping, the enhancement of renin-angiotensin system, and the expression of sympathetic nervous system or vasopressin work to balance the change, so

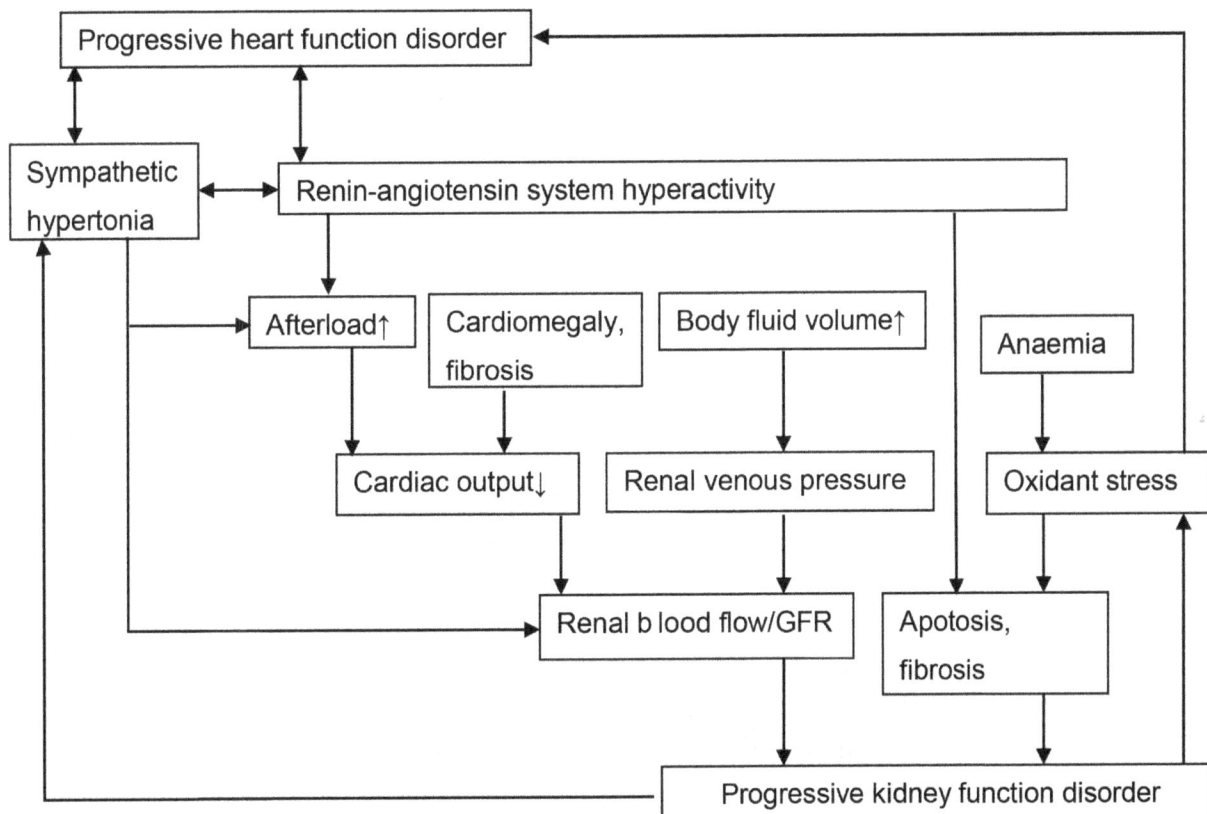

Figure 1. Correlation between heart function disorder and kidney function disorder.

blood pressure increases. However, with further progression of hepatic cirrhosis, the so-called cirrhosis cardiomyopathy occurs, and cardiac output is reduced by the reduction of myocardial extension ability and abnormality in the impulse conducting system [27]. In addition, cirrhosis is often associated with the development of comparative adrenal failure and has the tendency to reduce the blood pressure. To compensate, the renin-angiotensin system and the secretion of vasopressin are further increased [28]. Disorders in which free water cannot be drained from the kidney tubule or sodium retention is elevated cause sympathetic hyperactivity; as a result, circulating plasma volume cannot be reduced, leading to excess fluid accumulation as ascitic fluid or edema and hyponatremia [29]. In addition, sympathetic hyperactivity and vasopressin are vasoconstrictive, and renal blood flow is additionally reduced [25]. In other words, compensation, which was useful to maintain body blood pressure in the early onset of hepatic cirrhosis, reduces renal blood flow and leads to auto-regulation breakdown, inasmuch as it reduces glomerular filtration. Moreover, in cases of hepatic cirrhosis, even where there are no obvious infectious diseases, inflammatory cytokines, such as IL-6 or TNF-α, are elevated, and an impact for portal hypertension and circulation dynamics is considered [30].

3.2.2. Classification of clinical entity in hepatorenal syndrome

In general, hepatorenal syndrome, pathophysiologically, is broadly separated into two categories by the speed of progress of kidney function disorder. Quick progression (type 1) is defined as a serum creatinine level that is elevated more than two times within 2 weeks and elevated to more than 2.5 mg/dl; cases that progress more slowly are type 2. Part of the reason for classifying in this way is that type 1 is associated with singularly poor prognosis. The 3-month mortality rate of type 1 is almost 70%, while that of type 2 is approximately 10%, and it is reported that the median survival time after the onset of type 1 is approximately 2 weeks [31]. Some cases of type 1 involve a natural outbreak that develops into infections, such as spontaneous bacterial peritonitis, pneumonia, and opportunistic urinary tract infections [32, 33]. Therefore, early diagnosis and therapeutic intervention are desirable in type 1.

3.2.3. Diagnosis of hepatorenal syndrome

For diagnosis, the criterion of hepatorenal syndrome that has been traditionally propounded indicates that serum creatinine levels are elevated to more than 1.5 mg/dl [34]. That is, the condition requires that the serum creatinine level was more than 1.5 mg/dl in hepatorenal syndrome, regardless of the baseline level of hepatorenal syndrome or elevation degree and speed. This was viewed with suspicion in distinguishing AKI from CKD [35]. Then, ICA proposed a partial change of the diagnostic criteria for KDIGO, as AKI in hepatorenal syndrome patients, under the guidelines for AKI, which were announced by KDIGO and universally recognized. The difference in diagnostic criteria between ICA and KDIGO is the urinary output cut-off. The reason is that regardless of the relative maintenance of GFR, compared to other AKI, the potential for oliguria in hepatic cirrhosis patients is not negligible [11]. The ICA proposed to set the serum creatinine level within 3 months before admission as baseline, unless serum creatinine had been measured within the previous 7 days [35].

3.3. External injury and AKI

We give an outline of rhabdomyolysis (crush syndrome) in order to understand AKI due to external injury. Crush syndrome is a generalized diagnosis of the symptoms caused by skeletal muscle damage by external or other mechanical injury. First, regional edema occurs in the damaged skeletal muscle of the extremity, so that intravascular volume is reduced. Because the extremity compartment is restricted in space, the inner pressure of the compartment increases exponentially, and this in turn reduces arterial perfusion to the muscle. On the grounds that perfusion pressure is defined by the mean arterial blood pressure and compartment inner pressure, the perfusion pressure is conspicuously reduced under these circumstances, which means arterial blood pressure is low and compartment inner pressure is high. Skeletal muscle cells are destroyed by direct external or ischemic injury, and the intracellular components, including myoglobin, potassium, and urinary acid, are released and circulate at the time of reperfusion [36]. The mechanism of AKI by rhabdomyolysis remains to be explained; however, it is thought that it concerns the constriction of renal blood vessels directly, or ischemic renal tubular injury and tubular obstruction. Many different mechanisms have been related to the renovascular contraction characteristic of AKI by rhabdomyolysis. First, intravascular volume reduces in order to move fluid for the damaged skeletal muscle, and the renin-angiotensin system, vasopressin, or sympathetic nervous system cause hyperactivity, so kidney blood vessels contract. Next, increased levels of vascular mediators such as endothelin-1, thromboxane A2, TNF-α, and F2-isoprostane are additionally vasoconstrictive. Conversely, vasoactive nitric oxide (NO) is used to remove myoglobin such that a deficiency develops and renal blood flow becomes further diminished. Finally, a direct disorder caused by inflammation or oxidation with vascular endothelial disorder exacerbates these vascular mediators at the same time [37]. AKI by crush syndrome is also linked to the possibility of the same kidney disorder mechanism that occurs in tumor lysis syndrome, in addition to the mechanism of AKI by rhabdomyolysis described earlier, that is, a large amount of urinary acid being released from the injured skeletal muscle [38]. AKI by crush syndrome is more associated with the development of fluid overload, life-threatening acidosis, and hyperkalemia than AKI of other causes. Notably, an abrupt increase in potassium level, even if it remains within normal range, is an indication for dialysis [39, 40]. The dialysis initiation standards for AKI, especially dialysis initiation in an early period, remain greatly debated even though a large-scale trial has been conducted in recent years [41]. The evidence supporting renal replacement therapy for AKI caused by crush syndrome is limited and thus remains inconclusive. However, given that the high dialysis enforcement rate and clinical indications for fundamental therapy itself do not exist, early introduction may be useful [42]. Nevertheless, we should consider not only renal replacement therapy intended for the removal of myoglobin but also early introduction as for AKI [43].

3.4. Sepsis-associated AKI: SA-AKI

3.4.1. Mechanism of development and pathophysiology in SA-AKI

An "inflammation" mechanism is responsible for a large part of the occurrence of SA-AKI. When excessive inflammation is induced, organ damage is caused by hypercytokinemia, called a cytokine storm. For example, in endotoxemia caused by Gram-negative bacteria infection, the signal is released via Toll-like receptor (TLR) 4, mediators such as cytokines are released via the MyD88-dependent pathway or TRIF-dependent pathway, and factors promoting adherence to vascular endothelium are produced. Furthermore, in the glomerulus, expanding of the efferent arteriole, changes in tubuloglomerular feedback, and intumescence of the vascular endothelia are induced and result in a reduction of GFR. Furthermore, impaired renal tubular reabsorption of solutes or anaerobic metabolism by mitochondria occurs, and renal tubular dysfunction is caused by hypoxia of the medulla renalis [44]. However, in mice deficient in TLR4, which recognizes the endotoxin, and administered LPS organ-protection, action was not exhibited. In mice deficient in MyD88, which lies downstream of TLR4 [45], or TLR9, which recognizes bacterial DNA, AKI was alleviated [46]. This phenomenon can also be induced by other Gram-positive bacteria or viruses. Furthermore, when Bellomo et al. [47] measured renal blood flow in a sheep model with continuous infusion of bacteria, during hyperdynamic shock, which dilates peripheral blood vessels and increases cardiac output, renal blood flow increased, but glomerular filtration rate decreased. The cause was thought to be that the afferent arteriole dilated but the efferent arteriolar dilated without constriction. Progress of clinical condition additionally induces microvascular injury, which in turn induces afferent arteriole constriction and results in the persistent loss of glomerular filtration.

3.4.2. Risk factors

Risk factors of abnormal balance of tonus in the afferent/efferent, which is recognized in SA-AKI, include older age, preexisting chronic kidney disease (CKD) or cardiovascular condition, severe arteriosclerosis (hypertension, diabetes mellitus), and drug use (especially Ras inhibitors or NSAIDs).

3.4.3. Targeted therapy

Even though life-saving guidelines for sepsis treatment were proposed and practically applied, the incidence and severity of SA-AKI have not been alleviated [48]. The immediate action for patients with AKI is emergency response associated with severe kidney injury represented by severe uremia, hyperkalemia, volume overload (renal failure), or metabolic acidosis. When sepsis occurs, because of the relative lack of volume flow through the circulation, correcting volume flow through the circulation and maintaining perfusion rate of the kidney early are important. On the other hand, because excessive volume administration cannot improve circulatory dynamics and may worsen prognosis, vasoconstricting drugs should be administered after correcting volume flow through the circulation. With regard to the quality of transfusion, because artificial colloid solutions such as HES may cause further kidney injury in patients requiring renal replacement therapy (RRT) compared to extracellular fluids such as saline, their use should be avoided (VISEP study 2008, 6S trial 2012, CHEST study 2012). In the case that hyperdynamic shock occurs, to maintain organ perfusion pressure more than 65 mmHg, a vasoconstrictor drug (noradrenaline: NA) [49] is recommended as the first-line therapy, and vasopressin (VSP) is recommended as the second-line therapy. Furthermore, the focus of infection should be managed by drainage and so on. Antibacterial drugs should be administered as soon as possible, and if possible, injection with broad-spectrum antibiotics should be performed within an hour. At this time, antibiotics should be selected considering renal prognosis.

4. Prognosis of AKI

Studies on the long-term prognosis of AKI have advanced rapidly since approximately 2010 [50–62]. Consequently, advances in the understanding about the association between AKI and cardiovascular disturbance have been seen. The absence of consensus on the definition of recovery from AKI was previously considered problematic [63], and this problem was highlighted again by Sawhney's systematic review [61]. After this systematic review, two large studies, which were likely to be underpinnings of the consensus on the definition of recovery from AKI, were published [64, 65]. Accordingly, the importance of considering the time from the peak of SCr value to recovery and the importance of considering rehospitalization after recovery from AKI were suggested in order to define recovery from AKI. Although AKI or recovery from AKI was defined by SCr in all the above studies, it is impossible to capture changes in the tissues not reflected in kidney function because SCr value is the index of kidney function, and it is possible that changes in the kidney reflected in urine biomarkers have an impact on the long-term prognosis of AKI, even if there is no rise of SCr suggested, according to the article of the TRIBE-AKI study team [66]. It is necessary to think about what we can do for patients with AKI, and in the Japanese guidelines, it is recommended to assess the presence of a transition from AKI to CKD according to KDIGO guidelines. However, giving a referral for follow-up to patients targeted with clinical stratification stage 2 or stage 3, an outpatient department of a facility in Canada suggested, is because doing for patients with AKI includes those at clinical stratification stage 1 (in particular, the rise of SCr 0.3 mg/dl) is not realistic [67]. In actuality, in data from a US veteran's hospital in 2012, the rate of referral, even for patients at clinical stratification stage 2 or 3, to the department of internal nephrology medicine after discharge from a hospital is approximately 20%, and room for improvement was suggested [68]. Among patients with AKI receiving acute renal replacement therapy, there is evidence to suggest that there is a decreased mortality rate for patients who receive follow-up from a kidney physician [69]; it is possible that this outcome is attributable to the careful management by doctors whose reasons have not been considered. There is also an example of outcomes being improved when patients visit a doctor who conducts daily practice, even without a follow-up by a kidney physician [70]. There are data from the US that hospital physicians did not fully inform outpatient doctors during hospitalization for AKI onset [71]. It may be the role of the doctor who diagnosed AKI to inform the outpatient clinician of the risk of CKD onset and progression and avoiding prescription of drugs with renal toxicity after AKI.

Acknowledgements

We are grateful to Ms. Iku Niinomi, Mr. Yasuhiro Mori, and Mr. Yuki Yamaguchi for their assistance.

Conflict of interest

None.

Author details

Keiko Hosohata*, Ayaka Inada, Saki Oyama and Kazunori Iwanaga

*Address all correspondence to: hosohata@gly.oups.ac.jp

Education and Research Center for Clinical Pharmacy, Osaka University of Pharmaceutical Sciences, Takatsuki, Osaka, Japan

References

[1] Summary of recommendation statements. Kidney International. Supplement. 2012;**2**:8-12

[2] Bellomo R, Ronco C, Kellum JA, et al. Acute renal failure-definition, outcome measures, animal models, fluid therapy and information technology need: The second international consensus conference of the acute dialysis quality initiative(ADQI) group. Critical Care. 2004;**8**:R204-R212

[3] Kellum JA et al. Developing a consensus classification system for acute renal failure. Current Opinion in Critical Care. 2002;**8**:509-514

[4] Mehta RL, Kellum JA, Shah SV, et al. Acute Kidney Injury Network: Report of an initiative to improve outcomes in acute kidney injury. Critical Care. 2007;**11**:R31

[5] KDIGO. Clinical practice guideline for acute kidney injury. Nephron. Clinical Practice. 2012;**120**:c179-c184

[6] Rahman M, Shad F, Smith MC. Acute kidney injury: A guide to diagnosis and management. American Family Physician. 2012;**86**:631-639

[7] Eremina V, Jefferson JA, Kowalewska J, et al. VEGF inhibition and renal thrombotic microangiopathy. The New England Journal of Medicine. 2008;**358**:1129-1136

[8] Elyasi S, Khalili H, Dashti-Khavidaki S, et al. Vancomycin-induced nephrotoxicity: Mechanism, incidence, risk factors and special populations. A literature review. European Journal of Clinical Pharmacology. 2012;**68**:1243-1255

[9] Luque Y, Louis K, Jouanneau C, et al. Vancomycin-associated cast nephropathy. Journal of the American Society of Nephrology. 2017;**28**:1723-1728

[10] Markowitz GS, Nasr SH, Stokes MB, et al. Treatment with IFN-α, -β, or -γ is associated with collapsing focal segmental glomerulosclerosis. Clinical Journal of the American Society of Nephrology. 2010;**5**:607-615

[11] Nicola R, Shaqdan KW, Aran K, et al. Contrast-induced nephropathy: Identifying the risks, choosing the right agent, and reviewing effective prevention and management methods. Current Problems in Diagnostic Radiology. 2015;**44**:501-504

[12] Kanda T, Ishii K, Kawaguchi H, et al. High signal intensity in the dentate nucleus and globus pallidus on unenhanced T1-weighted MR images: Relationship with increasing cumulative dose of a gadolinium-based contrast material. Radiology. 2014;**270**:834-841

[13] Radbruch A. Are some agents less likely to deposit gadolinium in the brain? Magnetic Resonance Imaging. 2016;**34**:1351-1354

[14] Kartamihardja AA, Nakajima T, Kameo S, et al. Distribution and clearance of retained gadolinium in the brain: Differences between linear and macrocyclic gadolinium based contrast agents in a mouse model. The British Journal of Radiology. 2016;**89**:20160509

[15] Kartamihardja AA, Nakajima T, Kameo S, et al. Impact of impaired renal function on gadolinium retention after administration of gadolinium-based contrast agents in a mouse model. Investigative Radiology. 2016;**51**:655-660

[16] McDonald RJ, McDonald JS, Kallmes DF, et al. Gadolinium deposition in human brain tissues after contrast-enhanced MR imaging in adult patients without intracranial abnormalities. Radiology. 2017;**285**:546-554

[17] Hao D et al. MRI contrast agents: Basic chemistry and safety. Journal of Magnetic Resonance Imaging. 2012;**36**:1060-1071

[18] Brodsky SV, Nadasdy T, Rovin BH, et al. Warfarin-related nephropathy occurs in patients with and without chronic kidney disease and is associated with an increased mortality rate. Kidney International. 2011;**80**:181-189

[19] Ruffing KA, Hoppes P, Blend D. et al, Eosinophils in urine revisited. Clinical Nephrology. 1994;**41**:163-166

[20] Gonzalez E, Gutiérrez E, Galeano C, et al. Early steroid treatment improves the recovery of renal function in patients with drug-induced acute interstitial nephritis. Kidney International. 2008;**73**:940-946

[21] Bock JS et al. Cardiorenal syndrome new perspectives. Circulation. 2010;**121**:2592-2600

[22] Uchino S, Kellum JA, Bellomo R, et al. Acute renal failure in critically ill patients: A multinational, multicenter study. JAMA. 2005;**294**:813-818

[23] Heywood JT, Fonarow GC, Costanzo MR, et al. High prevalence of renal dysfunction and its impact on outcome in 118,465 patients hospitalized with acute decompensated heart failure: A report from the ADHERE database. Journal of Cardiac Failure. 2007;**13**:422-430

[24] Ronco C, McCullough P, Anker SD, et al. Cardiorenal syndromes: Report from the consensus conference of the acute dialysis quality initiative. European Heart Journal. 2010;**31**:703-711

[25] Durand F, Graupera I, Gines P, et al. Pathogenesis of hepatorenal syndrome: Implications for therapy. American Journal of Kidney Diseases. 2016;**67**:318-328

[26] Bolognesi M, Di Pascoli M, Verardo A, et al. Splanchnic vasodilation and hyperdynamic circulatory syndrome in cirrhosis. World Journal of Gastroenterology. 2014;**20**:2555-2563

[27] Ruiz-del-Arbal L, Serradilla R. Cirrhotic cardiomyopathy. World Journal of Gastroen-terology. 2015;**21**:11502-11521

[28] Karagiannis AK, Nakouti T, Pipili C, et al. Adrenal insufficiency in patients with decom-pensated cirrhosis. World Journal of Hepatology. 2015;**7**:1112-1124

[29] John S, Thuluvath PJ. Hyponatremia in cirrhosis: Pathophysiology and management. World Journal of Gastroenterology. 2015;**21**:3197-3205

[30] Dirchwolf M, Ruf AE. Role of systemic inflammation in cirrhosis:From pathogenesis to prognosis. World Journal of Hepatology. 2015;**7**:1974-1981

[31] Gines P, Guevara M, Arroyo V, et al. Hepatorenal syndrome. Lancet. 2003;**362**:1819-1827

[32] Fasolato S, Angeli P, Dallagnese L, et al. Renal failure and bacterial infections in patients with cirrhosis: Epidemiology and clinical features. Hepatology (Baltimore). 2007; **45**:223-229

[33] Baraldi O, Valentini C, Donati G, et al. Hepatorenal syndrome: Update on diagnosis and treatment. World Journal of Nephrology. 2015;**4**:511-520

[34] Salerno F, Gerbes A, Gines P, et al. Diagnosis, prevention and treatment of hepatorenal syndrome in cirrhosis. Gut. 2007;**56**:1310-1318

[35] Angeli P, Gines P, Wong F, et al. Diagnosis and management of acute kidney injury in patients with cirrhosis:Revised consensus recommendations of the International Club of Ascites. Journal of Hepatology. 2015;**62**:968-974

[36] Gibney RT, Sever MS, Vanholder RC. Disaster nephrology:Crush injury and beyond. Kidney International. 2014;**85**:1049-1057

[37] Bosch X, Poch E, Grau JM. Rhabdomyolysis and acute kidney injury. The New England Journal of Medicine. 2009;**361**:62-72

[38] Chavez LO, Leon M, EinaV S, et al. Beyond muscle destruction: A systematic review of rhabdomyolysis for clinical practice. Critical Care. 2016;**20**:135

[39] Sever MS, Vanholder R, RDRTF of ISN Work Group on Recommendations for the Management of Crush Victims in Mass Disasters. Recommendation for the management of crush victims in mass disasters. Nephrology, Dialysis, Transplantation. 2012;**27**(Suppl 1):i1-i67

[40] Sever MS, Erek E, Vanholder R, et al. Serum potassium in the crush syndrome victims of the Marmara disaster. Clinical Nephrology. 2003;**59**:326-333

[41] Bagshaw SM, Wald R. Strategies for the optimal timing to start renal replacement therapy in critically ill patients with acute kidney injury. Kidney International. 2017;**91**:1022-1032

[42] Sever MS, Vanholder R. Management of crush victims in mass disasters: Highlights from recently published recommendations. Clinical Journal of the American Society of Nephrology. 2013;**8**:328-335

[43] Petejova N, Martinek A. Acute kidney injury due to rhabdomyolysis and renal replacement therapy: A critical review. Critical Care. 2014;**18**:224

[44] Anderberg SB, Luther T, Frithiof R, et al. Physiological aspects of toll-like receptor 4 activation in sepsis-induced acute kidney injury. Acta Physiologica. 2017;**219**:573-588

[45] Dear JW, Yasuda H, Hu X, et al. Sepsis-induced organ failure is mediated by different pathways in the kidney and liver: Acute renal failure is dependent on MyD88 but not renal cell apoptosis. Kidney International. 2006;**69**:832-836

[46] Yasuda H, Leelahavanichkul A, Tsunoda S, et al. Chloroquine and inhibition of toll-like receptor 9 protect from sepsis-induced acute kidney injury. American Journal of Physiology. Renal Physiology. 2008;**294**:F1050-F1058

[47] Prowle JR, Bellomo R. Sepsis-associated acute kidney injury: Macrohemodynamic and microhemodynamic alterations in the renal circulation. Seminars in Nephrology. 2015;**35**:64-74

[48] Ahmed W, Memon JI, Rehmani R, et al. Outcome of patients with acute kidney injury in severe sepsis and septic shock treated with early goal-directed therapy in an intensive care unit. Saudi Journal of Kidney Diseases and Transplantation. 2014;**25**:544-551

[49] Albanèse J, Leone M, Garnier F, et al. Renal effects of norepinephrine in septic and non-septic patients. Chest. 2004;**126**:534-539

[50] Flynn JT. Choice of dialysis modality for management of pediatric acute renal failure. Pediatric Nephrology. 2002;**17**:61-69

[51] Kaddourah A, Basu RK, Bagshaw SM, et al. Epidemiology of acute kidney injury in critically ill children and young adults. The New England Journal of Medicine. 2017;**376**:11-20

[52] Barbour T, Johnson S, Cohney S, et al. Thrombotic microangiopathy and associated renal disorders. Nephrology, Dialysis, Transplantation. 2012;**27**:2673-2685

[53] Besbas N, Karpman D, Landau D, et al. European Paediatric research group for HUS: A classification of hemolytic uremic syndrome and thrombotic thrombocytopenic purpura and related disorders. Kidney International. 2006;**70**:423-431

[54] Scully M, Goodship T. How I treat thrombotic thrombocytopenic purpura and atypical haemolytic uraemic syndrome. British Journal of Haematology. 2014;**164**:759-766

[55] George JN, Nester CM. Syndromes of thrombotic microangiopathy. The New England Journal of Medicine. 2014;**371**:654-666

[56] Loirat C, Fakhouri F, Ariceta G, et al. An international consensus approach to the management of atypical hemolytic uremic syndrome in children. Pediatric Nephrology. 2016;**31**:15-39

[57] Noris M, Remuzzi G. Atypical hemolytic-uremic syndrome. The New England Journal of Medicine. 2009;**361**:1676-1687

[58] Greenberg JH, Parikh CR. Biomarkers for diagnosis and prognosis of AKI in children: One size does not fit all. Clinical Journal of the American Society of Nephrology. 2017; **12**:1551-1557

[59] Coca SG, Yusuf B, Shlipak MG, et al. Long-term risk of mortality and other adverse outcomes after acute kidney injury: A systematic review and meta-analysis. American Journal of Kidney Diseases. 2009;**53**:961-973

[60] Coca SG, Singanamala S, Parikh CR. Chronic kidney disease after acute kidney injury: A systematic review and meta-analysis. Kidney International. 2012;**81**:442-448

[61] Sawwhney S, Mitchell M, Marks A, et al. Long-term prognosis after acute kidney injury (AKI): What is the role of baseline kidney function and recovery? A systematic review. BMJ Open. 2015;**5**:e006497

[62] Odutayo A, Wong CX, Farkouh M, et al. AKI and long-term risk for cardiovascular events and mortality. Journal of the American Society of Nephrology. 2017;**28**:377-387

[63] Kellum JA. How can we define recovery after acute kidney injury? Considerations from epidemiology and clinical trial design. Nephron. Clinical Practice. 2014;**127**:81-88

[64] Heung M, Steffic DE, Zivin K, et al. Acute kidney injury recovery pattern and subsequent risk of CKD: An analysis of veterans health administration data. American Journal of Kidney Diseases. 2016;**67**:742-752

[65] Kellum JA, Sileanu FE, Bihorac A, et al. Recovery after kidney injury. American Journal of Respiratory and Critical Care Medicine. 2017;**195**:784-791

[66] Coca SG, Garg AX, Thiessen-Philbrook H, et al. Urinary biomarkers of AKI and mortality 3 years after cardiac surgery. Journal of the American Society of Nephrology. 2014;**25**:1063-1071

[67] Silver SA, Goldstein SL, Harel Z, et al. Ambulatory care after acute kidney injury: An opportunity to improve patient outcomes. Canadian Journal of Kidney Health and Disease. 2015;**2**(36)

[68] Siew ED, Petrson JF, Eden SK, et al. Outpatient nephrology referral rates after acute kidney injury. Journal of the American Society of Nephrology. 2012;**23**:305-312

[69] Harel Z, Wald R, Bargman JM, et al. Nephrologist follow-up improves all-cause mortality of severe acute kidney injury survivors. Kidney International. 2013;**83**:901-908

[70] Lipworth L, Abdel-Kader K, Morse J, et al. High prevalence of non-steroidal anti-inflammatory drug use among acute kidney injury survivors in the southern community cohort study. BMC Nephrology. 2016;**17**(189)

[71] Greer RC, Liu Y, Crews DC, et al. Hospital discharge communications during care transitions for patients with acute kidney injury: A cross-sectional study. BMC Health Services Research. 2016;**16**(449)

2

New Tubulocentric Insights for Diabetic Nephropathy: From Pathophysiology to Treatment

Sang Soo Kim, Jong Ho Kim, Su Mi Lee,
Il Young Kim and Sang Heon Song

Abstract

The prevalence of diabetes is increasing worldwide, and one of the most important complications, diabetic nephropathy, constitutes a significant global health care and socioeconomic burden. Glomerular dysfunction is a major factor in the development and progression of diabetic nephropathy. However, emerging evidence suggests that tubular damage also plays an important role in the pathogenesis of diabetic nephropathy. This tubulocentric view shifts the focus markedly from glomeruli to proximal tubules, which might have an important role as a trigger or a driver in the early development and progression of diabetic nephropathy. Accordingly, numerous studies have focused on several different tubular damage markers that are clinically indicated as potential biomarkers for the early detection of diabetic nephropathy. Furthermore, these findings are relevant for identifying therapeutics for diabetic nephropathy that target the proximal tubules. This review outlines new tubulocentric insights into diabetic nephropathy, from pathophysiological mechanisms to diagnostic and therapeutic approaches.

Keywords: biomarkers, diabetic nephropathy, glomerulus, proximal tubules, SGLT2 inhibitors

1. Introduction

Diabetes is often accompanied by chronic kidney disease (CKD) and accounts for more than half of the cause of end-stage renal disease (ESRD) and dialysis [1]. With the increasing prevalence of diabetes and high morbidity and mortality, its complications such as diabetic nephropathy impose great burden on individuals with diabetes and their society as well [2]. It is unclear whether the glomerulus or tubules are more important in the development and progression of diabetic nephropathy. The phenomenon of glomerulosclerosis led to an interest in the glomerulus as the primary site of injury in diabetic nephropathy. Indeed, changes in glomerular structure, such as glomerular basement membrane thickening, mesangial expansion, and nodular/global glomerulosclerosis, are key findings for the diagnosis of diabetic nephropathy and other forms of glomerulonephropathy [3]. Although changes in the glomerulus in diabetic neuropathy undoubtedly occur, there is growing evidence to suggest a prominent role for the proximal tubules as triggers or drivers of diabetic nephropathy. Indeed, this evidence provides a new perspective on the natural course and pathophysiology of diabetic nephropathy. These novel insights also provide new opportunities for diagnostic and therapeutic progress through targeting the proximal tubules in diabetic nephropathy. This review provides an outline of diabetic nephropathy, from the underlying pathophysiological mechanism to diagnostic and therapeutic approaches, based on a tubulocentric perspective.

2. Natural course of diabetic nephropathy: old and new

It is very important to understand the natural course of disease to ensure that technical advances are fully exploited. However, the natural course of diabetic nephropathy is complex and depends on several factors, such as the clinical treatments used, and the race, type of diabetes, and comorbidities of the patient. Therefore, it is difficult to treat and prevent diabetic nephropathy. Current treatments include renin-angiotensin system (RAS) blockade, antihypertensives, glycemic control, and correction of dyslipidemia for the management of diabetic complications. Diabetes mellitus (DM) has a long history and was first described in 1552 BC; it has long been recognized as a socioeconomic burden [4]. Diabetes is regarded as a metabolic derangement and is closely related to renal dysfunction, as a microvascular complication [5]. Classically, diabetic nephropathy has a five-stage natural history: hyperfiltration, silent nephropathy, incipient nephropathy (microalbuminuric stage), overt nephropathy (macroalbuminuric stage), and ESRD [6, 7]. These five stages are almost exclusively applied to discussions of type 1 diabetes since the precise onset of disease in type 2 diabetes is not known. This natural course of diabetic nephropathy has served as a basis for clinical practice, and there are ongoing efforts to reduce albuminuria in patients with type 2 diabetes and renal dysfunction. Most adult cases of diabetes are type 2, and it is critical to delineate the progress of this disease. Type 2 diabetes differs from type 1 diabetes in several aspects. First, it is impossible to determine disease onset in type 2 diabetes. Second, in many cases, hypertension and albuminuria commonly accompany type 2 diabetes. Third, microalbuminuria has a lower predictive value for renal dysfunction because of the high mortality rate caused by cardiovascular disease [7, 8]. Recently, a new paradigm was suggested for exploring the natural course of diabetic nephropathy in the context of microalbuminuria and the nonclassical form of the disease.

2.1. Microalbuminuria: moderately increased albuminuria

Microalbuminuria is a robust indicator of the onset and progression of diabetic nephropathy, and it is assessed by reference to serum creatinine levels or the estimated glomerular filtration rate (eGFR). However, microalbuminuria has some major limitations as a predictor of renal dysfunction [9]. Albuminuria measurements can be imprecise and vary widely according to the assay method used, the time of urine collection, and the presence of clinical conditions such as fever, urinary tract infection, and congestive heart failure, as well as by exercise status [10]. Microalbuminuria was originally considered a subcategory denoted by an albuminuria level of 30–299 mg/day in a 24-h urine sample or 30–299 mg/g creatinine in a spot urine sample. Recently, normoalbuminuria and microalbuminuria were replaced by "normal to mildly increased albuminuria" and "moderately increased albuminuria," respectively, because albuminuria is directly related to all-cause mortality, cardiovascular mortality, and renal dysfunction, even in patients with normoalbuminuria and microalbuminuria [11, 12] Furthermore, microalbuminuria shows dynamic characteristics (**Figure 1**), being a transient state that can progress to macroalbuminuria or regress to normoalbuminuria [13, 14]. A 7-year prospective study performed by the EURODIAB IDDM Complications Study Group in 352 type 1 diabetic patients showed that ~14% progressed to macroalbuminuria, 35% remained in a microalbuminuric state, and 51% regressed to normoalbuminuria [13]. The Joslin study reported that 58% of 386 type 1 diabetic patients with persistent microalbuminuria regressed to normoalbuminuria [14]. A better glycemic control contributes to the regression of microalbuminuria, and almost half of patients with microalbuminuria can regress to normoalbuminuria, as evidenced by the above two large studies. Although microalbuminuria is caused by glomerular injury, recent research has focused on the role of tubular dysfunction in albuminuria in type 1 diabetes. The Second Joslin Kidney Study reported that kidney injury molecule-1 (KIM-1) and N-acetyl-β-D-glucosaminidase (NAG) levels were important for predicting the regression of microalbuminuria [15]. This finding supports the theory that tubular injury plays a significant role in the progression of renal complications in type 1 diabetes. This pattern of microalbuminuria regression could also be applicable to type 2 diabetes, although no concrete evidence for this has been reported.

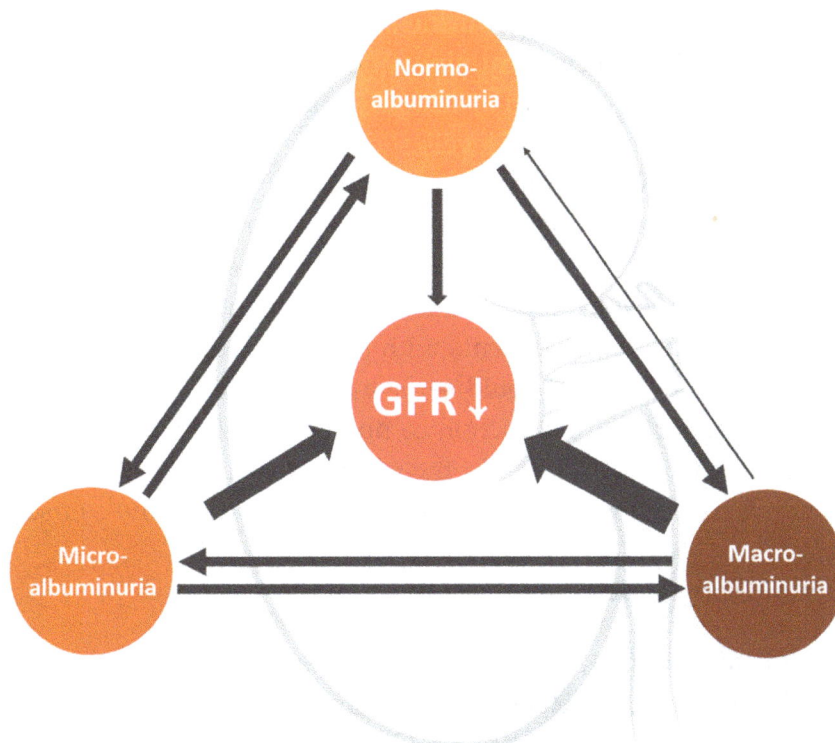

Figure 1. A triangle concept toward kidney function. eGFR, estimated glomerular filtration rate.

In 216 Japanese patients with type 2 diabetes and microalbuminuria, the regression rate to a normoalbuminuric state was ~50%, where regression was associated with a RAS-blocking agent, a better glycemic control, and a tight control of blood pressure [9]. However, none of 60 patients with type 2 microalbuminuric diabetic nephropathy regressed to normoalbuminuria in an African-American population [16]. This suggests that there are racial differences in changes in microalbuminuria status in type 2 diabetes, and further studies are needed to explore the role of genetic predisposition and race. A recent study suggested that macroalbuminuria and microalbuminuria can regress to microalbuminuria or normoalbuminuria, respectively [17]. In the FinnDiane study, 23.4% of 475 type 1 diabetic patients with macroalbuminuria regressed to a lower categorical albuminuric state and 2.5% regressed to normoalbuminuria, although the statistical power was low [17]. Such regression would improve the cardiovascular prognosis and all-cause mortality. Previous studies proposed that the regression of microalbuminuria contributes to a reduction in renal or cardiovascular risk in type 2 diabetic and hypertensive patients [18, 19]. These data suggest that it is necessary to treat diabetic patients with some degree of albuminuria to regress the albuminuria.

2.2. Nonalbumin proteinuria

Protein in urine comprises albumin (40%) and nonalbumin proteins (NAPs; 60%). A third of NAPs are low-molecular weight proteins (LMWP), such as light-chain immunoglobulins (20%), and two-thirds are Tamm-Horsfall mucoproteins produced by the distal tubules [20, 21]. The proportional contribution of albumin attributes to be largely more variable at lower levels of proteinuria, and NAPs are important when assessing proteinuria as a biomarker of renal tubular damage [22]. Nonalbumin proteinuria can be defined as an albumin excretion rate (AER) of < 30 mg/24 h with a protein excretion rate (PER) of >149 mg/24 h. Nonalbumin proteinuria can be quantified in random spot urine samples using the following formula: NAP-to-creatinine ratio (NAPCR) = protein creatinine ratio (PCR) − albumin creatinine ratio (ACR). Because albuminuria tests could miss up to 40% of females and 30.8% of males in the general population with gross proteinuria, NAP levels should be checked to accurately assess renal damage [21]. Our laboratory reported that urinary NAPCR had a significant association with the decline in eGFR of 237 type 2 diabetic patients with preserved kidney function and normoalbuminuria [23]. In addition, NAP was related to tubular biomarkers such as KIM-1, neutrophil gelatinase-associated lipocalin (NGAL), and liver-type fatty acid-binding protein (L-FABP) in early type 2 diabetic nephropathy patients with preserved kidney function (eGFR ≥60 mL/min/1.73 m²) [24]. Moreover, NAPCR could serve a simpler and a more practical marker for assessing the progression of renal dysfunction compared with laboratory urinary biomarkers, such as KIM-1, NGAL, and L-FABP [25]. In the future, it will be necessary to study NAP in diabetic nephropathy to discover novel processes in and investigate the course of the disease.

2.3. Normoalbuminuric renal decline (NARD)

In general clinical practice, the eGFR should be calculated at least once a year to properly manage diabetic patients. Like albuminuria, eGFR has some major limitations for predicting renal dysfunction, because serum creatinine and cystatin C levels cannot be measured precisely and do not reflect early changes in the kidney. However, currently, there are no available tools that are more powerful for assessing kidney function. Although the classic course of diabetic nephropathy involves sequential dysfunction of the kidney following albuminuria, recent epidemiologic data suggested the presence of normoalbuminuric diabetic nephropathy in some patients [26]. There is a close relationship between albuminuria and progressive dysfunction of the diabetic kidney. A recent Japanese study showed that a rapid decline in kidney function occurred in subjects with higher levels of ACR of ≥3000 mg/g creatinine in urine. In addition, the rate of annual decline in eGFR was doubled in macroalbuminuric versus normoalbuminuric diabetics for 9.2 years [11]. However, the focus should be on NARD with respect to early intervention strategies, because dipstick tests cannot reveal low levels of albuminuria or NAP. The UK Prospective Diabetes Study (UKPDS) reported that, among the patients who developed renal impairment during the study, 61% did not have albuminuria beforehand and 39% never developed albuminuria [27]. This suggests that distinct pathobiological mechanisms may underlie NARD and albuminuric renal decline. The prevalence of NARD was not low (20.5–63%) in several clinical trials performed in type 2 diabetic patients [26]. Interestingly, in another study, the prevalence of retinopathy was lower in the NARD group than in the albuminuric group, and patients with NARD had a shorter duration of diabetes [28]. This finding gives rise to a new hypothesis, in which NARD is not to be related to microangiopathy and instead shows a greater association with tubulointerstitial damage or macroangiopathy (i.e., arteriosclerosis).

Most diabetic patients with albuminuria show typical renal pathological changes, whereas typical diabetic glomerular changes are observed less frequently. In addition, atypical histologic changes suggestive of a severe interstitial or a tubular damage, or varying degrees of arteriosclerosis, were seen in patients with NARD [29]. Intrarenal arteriosclerosis is related to aging and hypertension. Furthermore, a recent study suggested that acute kidney injury (AKI) is a major component of CKD in patients with diabetes [30]. Both clinically evident and subclinical AKI can damage proximal tubular cells, podocytes, and endothelial cells, and such insults can create an apoptotic and inflammatory environment within the kidneys. Atubular glomeruli and glomerulotubular junction abnormalities in diabetes are also related to AKI and can lead to NARD [31].

2.4. Progressive renal decline (PRD)

Diabetic nephropathy has several phenotypes according to clinical and laboratory data; among them, PRD is the most serious. Generally, PRD is defined as a >3.5 mL/min/year loss in the eGFR in type 1 diabetes and PRD reasonably included NARD. Krolewski reported that the prevalence of PRD was 10, 32, and 50% in patients with normoalbuminuria, microalbuminuria, and macroalbuminuria, respectively [32]. The recent Scottish Go-DARTS study identified biomarkers for PRD: 154 patients with type 2 diabetes and CKD showed a >40% decline in eGFR during the 3.5-year study period [33]. In the second Joslin Kidney Study, in which PRD was defined as a decrease in eGFR >30% from baseline during ≤5 years of follow-up, an early decline in renal function developed in 6 and 18% of patients with normoalbuminuric and microalbuminuric diabetes, respectively [34]. Although the mechanism underlying such a decline is unclear, more intensive and personalized treatments are needed to prevent progression to ESRD.

The clinical course of diabetic nephropathy varies such that physicians should treat diabetic patients using tailored approaches; the term "natural course" may no longer be applicable in this era of active interventions. In future, more phenotype-specific approaches informed by gene- and proteome-based analyses are needed to improve patient prognosis.

3. Pathophysiology of diabetic nephropathy: tubule versus glomerulus

Glomerular dysfunction has long been considered a major driver of diabetic nephropathy. Kimmelstiel-Wilson nodules, which are characterized by the formation of diffuse nodular lesions of a pink hyaline material in glomerular capillary loops in the glomerulus [35], have contributed greatly to the identification of the glomerulus as the main culprit in the development of diabetic nephropathy. Diabetes-induced glomerulopathy can be caused by interactions among glomerular endothelial cells, mesangial cells, and podocytes via metabolic and hemodynamic perturbations [36]. However, glomerulopathy in diabetes is still not fully understood because various cells resident within the glomeruli have different roles in the disease process. Furthermore, recent studies revealed that glomerulopathy is preceded by tubular dysfunction during the development and progression of diabetic nephropathy [37]. These tubulocentric concept addressed in this chapter is summarized in **Figure 2**.

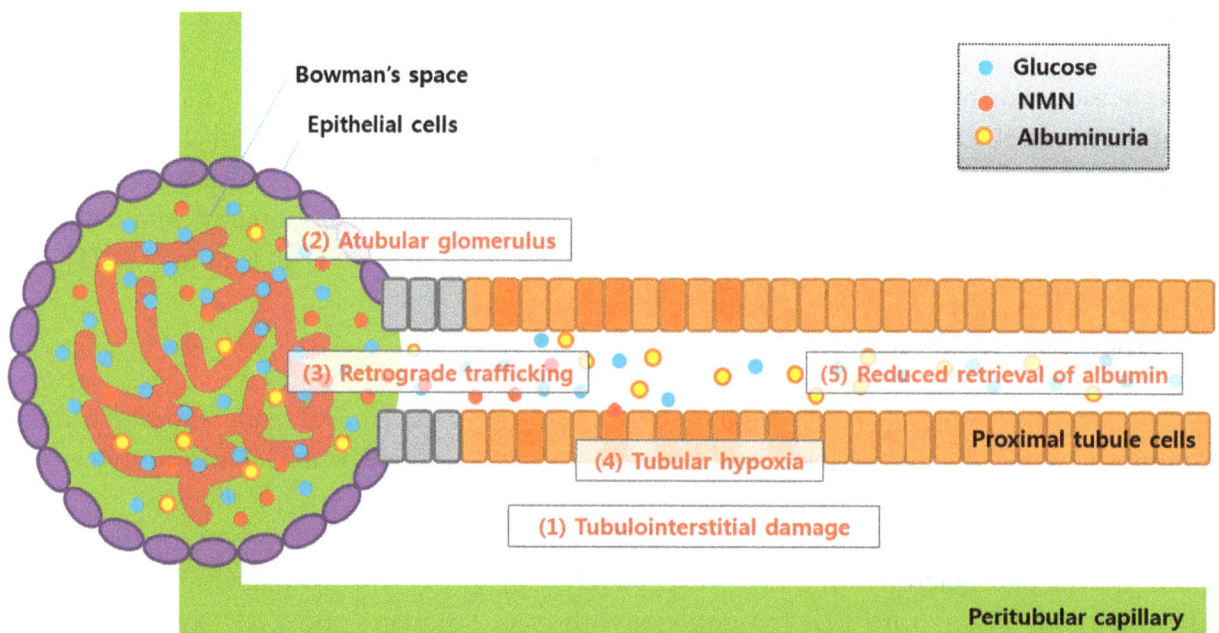

Figure 2. Tubulocentric concept for diabetic nephropathy. (1) Tubulointerstitial damage can cause a disconnect between glomerulus and tubule, (2) atubular glomerulus, (3) retrograde trafficking with NMN releasing by proximal tubule can contribute glomerulopathy, (4) proximal tubules are vulnerable to hypoxic injury, which can lead to fibrosis and apoptosis, (5) reduced retrieval of albumin by impaired tubule resorption is responsible for albuminuria in diabetic nephropathy.

3.1. Proximal tubules contribute to glomerulopathy

Pathological changes in the tubulointerstitium that have been linked to diabetic nephropathy include the thickening of the tubular basement membrane (TBM), tubular atrophy, interstitial fibrosis, and arteriosclerosis, which are closely correlated with the magnitude of renal dysfunction and albuminuria [38]. Furthermore, such tubulointerstitial damage can cause a disconnect between the glomerulus and the proximal tubule, the so-called atubular glomerulus, which is an important and a common cause of irreversible CKD progression [39, 40]. These glomerulotubular junction abnormalities accompanied by atubular glomerulus have been linked to the development and progression of diabetic nephropathy in both type 1 and 2 diabetes [31, 41]. Recent studies suggest that the glomerular dysfunction triggered by proximal tubules, the so-called retrograde trafficking might be important in diabetic nephropathy [42, 43]. Proximal tubules communicate with podocytes by releasing nicotinamide mononucleotide (NMN), and proximal tubule-specific Sirt1 protects against diabetic kidney disease by maintaining glomerular NMN concentrations and preserving podocyte function [42]. Furthermore, injured proximal tubule epithelium can trigger an inflammatory response, and repeated injury results in maladaptive repair. This in turn leads to tubulointerstitial fibrosis, tubular atrophy, and, potentially, secondary glomerulosclerosis, which is pathologically similar to classic diabetic nephropathy [44]. Albuminuria, which has been primarily considered as a glomerular damage marker, is a sensitive marker, reflecting the functional impairment in tubule, alone or in combination with glomerular origin in animal nephrotoxicity study [45]. Finally, a substantial evidence from human urinary biomarker data supports that proximal tubule damage might have an important role in the development of early diabetic nephropathy as a primary cause, not a secondary phenomenon [46].

3.2. Tubular hypoxia hypothesis

In diabetic kidney, proximal tubules are vulnerable to hypoxic injury because of an increased oxygen consumption, an impaired oxygen utilization, and a reduced oxygen delivery. Sodium reabsorption and gluconeogenesis processes occurring at the proximal tubules consume oxygen. The proximal tubule can be subdivided into three distinct segments (S1, S2, and S3) and is adapted for reabsorption. Transport across the tubular epithelium occurs via two routes: transcellular transport across luminal and basolateral membranes via Na^+, K^+ −adenosine triphosphatase (ATPase), and paracellular transport through tight junctions and the intercellular space. Glucose enters cells in the proximal tubule via the sodium-glucose cotransporter (SGLT), and is extruded from cells by GLUT1 and GLUT2 [47]. High Na^+, K^+-ATPase activity and oxygen consumption levels are needed to reabsorb glucose under high glucose conditions. A recent study showed that SGLT2 inhibitors downregulate Na^+ and K^+-ATPase activity and eventually reduce energy or oxygen requirements [48]. Similar to hepatocytes, epithelial cells in proximal tubules perform gluconeogenesis and export glucose into the circulation via oxygen- and energy-based processes. In diabetes, renal gluconeogenesis is particularly increased in the postprandial or fasting state [49]. Hypoxia induces apoptosis by upregulating Fas expression [50, 51]. Hypoxia stimulates extracellular matrix (ECM) expansion via transforming growth factor-β (TGF-β)-dependent and -independent pathways, such as an increased collagen production, a decreased matrix metalloproteinase-2 (MMP-2) activity, and an increased tissue inhibitor of metalloproteinase-1 (TIMP-1) expression [52, 53].

Recently, our laboratory studied the role of MMP-2 in diabetic nephropathy. Hyperglycemia-induced oxidative stress is a major driver of diabetic nephropathy, and high glucose levels stimulated the induction of intracellular MMP-2 in HK2 cells; this expression was blocked by the NF-κB inhibitor pyrrolidine dithiocarbamate (PDTC) [54]. Intracellular MMP-2 exacerbates oxidative stress by inducing the mitochondrial permeability transition, which results in tubular epithelial cell-regulated necrosis [55]. Therefore, intracellular MMP-2 is related to oxidative stress, and proximal tubular cells are susceptible to hypoxic stress. This may be important in the pathogenesis of CKD in DM. The resultant may lead to glomerular change as well as tubulointerstitial hypoxia and finally loss of kidney function.

3.3. Intermittent and continuous injurious stimuli lead to proximal tubulopathy and CKD

Unlike healthy individuals, patients with diabetes are persistently exposed to various metabolic and hemodynamic factors that sustain the disease state [56]. In addition, AKI frequently occurs after various nephrotoxic insults, such as ischemia during cardiac surgery and those associated with the administration of contrast media. The proximal tubule is particularly vulnerable to the ischemia and toxin-mediated injury that lead to AKI. In a mouse model of induced proximal tubule injury, tubular regeneration after a single episode of renal epithelium injury was robust and efficient, leading to complete restoration of the kidney architecture [45]. However, repeated injury resulted in maladaptive repair, manifested as tubulointerstitial fibrosis and tubular atrophy, and with the potential for secondary glomerulosclerosis [45]. Thus, these data suggest that the cumulative effects of repeated episodes of subclinical AKI arising from injurious stimuli lead to the progressive tubulointerstitial fibrosis that is characteristic of CKD, including diabetic nephropathy. Epidemiological and clinical observations support a relationship between intermittent AKI and CKD progression in diabetic patients [57, 58]. AKI increased the risk of advanced CDK in diabetic patients independent of other major risk factors of kidney disease progression, and each episode of AKI showed a cumulative dose-response association, doubling the risk of stage 4 CKD [57]. In AKI, a low eGFR and/or an elevated albuminuria level are compelling biomarkers for major adverse outcomes and death in diabetes [58].

3.4. Tubular contribution to albuminuria

The role of proximal tubules in albuminuria in various renal disorders, including diabetic nephropathy, remains controversial. The glomerular filtration barrier has long been considered largely impermeable to albumin, but recent data suggest that it may not be especially important in this process [59]. According to the "retrieval hypothesis," albuminuria likely has a tubular origin, because albumin can be filtered by normal glomeruli in the nephrotic range if tubular reabsorption is only partial [60, 61]. Russo et al. [60] reported that more albumin was filtered and underwent a rapid retrieval process via transcytosis in proximal tubule cells. Therefore, controversy remains regarding the extent of the glomerular filtration of albumin. A study of Fanconi syndrome patients with proteinuria reported a markedly impaired albumin filtration rate [62]. Collectively, these data suggest that an increased glomerular leakage and an impaired tubular reabsorption are not mutually incompatible, and both are accountable for albuminuria in the early diabetic nephropathy [61, 63].

4. Tubular biomarkers of diabetic nephropathy

Classification of diabetic nephropathy based on albuminuria and the eGFR provides prognostic information that is helpful to guide therapeutic decisions. Albuminuria serves as a marker of endothelial dysfunction, which is a prognostic factor for renal impairments and a high cardiovascular risk [64]. However, its progress is unpredictable, since microalbuminuria can regress toward normoalbuminuria, progress toward macroalbuminuria, or remain stable [65]. Moreover, diabetic nephropathy can develop in normoalbuminuric patients. In addition, structural changes in the glomerulus may appear before the onset of microalbuminuria, even though microalbuminuria is the established screening tool for diabetic nephropathy [66]. Therefore, an intensive search for new blood or urine biomarkers that could improve diagnostic and prognostic precision in diabetic nephropathy has recently been reported.

4.1. Classification

Because of emerging evidence supporting tubulocentric concepts in diabetic nephropathy, the focus has shifted from glomeruli to proximal tubules, which may contribute to the pathogenesis of diabetic nephropathy from an early stage. Both functional and structural markers can be used to detect proximal tubule dysfunction in diabetic nephropathy. One method is to detect filtered proteins due to the impaired reabsorption by the proximal tubules. The main site for reabsorbing filtered proteins is the proximal tubules and, assuming no secretion or degradation of these proteins through the glomerulus, the more proteins are filtered, the higher the urinary excretion rate will be when tubular reabsorption is destroyed. These functional tubular biomarkers are low-molecular weight proteins (LMWP) that are mostly reabsorbed by the proximal tubules. Another method is to detect proteins released into the urine by tubular injury. These urinary proteins are structural tubular biomarkers that come directly from tubular cells rather than from plasma. The principal tubular biomarkers in diabetic nephropathy are briefly described in **Table 1**.

4.2. Clinical utility

In tubular proteinuria, the endocytic function of proximal tubule is damaged and a large amount of LMWP is detected in the urine. For example, retinol-binding protein 4 is markedly elevated when endocytic function is completely eliminated [67]. The cause of an increased LMWP excretion in diabetes is usually explained by tubular disease. Animal models suggest the pathway that the filtered proteins compete with each other for reabsorption in proximal tubules [68]. Clinical studies have also shown that the same pathway leads to the reabsorption of albumin and LMWP through glomeruli [69]. The ability of protein reabsorption in proximal tubules is not known but competition for reabsorption between albumin and LMWP may occur. As a result, a slight increase in filtered albumin through glomeruli in the early stage of diabetic nephropathy will not cause albuminuria, but an increase in LMWP excretion may be detected indirectly. In other words, early glomerular injury in diabetes may not

Functional tubular biomarkers

Albumin	65 kDa	Normally filtered very little at the glomerulus. With glomerular barrier damage, filtration occurs and followed by tubular reabsorption. The resulting albuminuria reflects the combined contribution of these two processes.
Cystatin C	13 kDa	Filtered by the glomerulus and reabsorbed in the proximal tubule. No tubular secretion.
Retinol-binding protein 4	21 kDa	
α_1-microglobulin	26–31 kDa	
β_2-microglobulin	11.8 kDa	Filtered by the glomerulus and degraded in the proximal tubule via a megalin-dependent pathway. Unstable in urine.

Structural tubular biomarkers

Neutrophil gelatinase-associated lipocalin (NGAL)	25 kDa	Hyper-produced in the kidney tubules within a few hours after renal ischemia-reperfusion injury. It is freely filtered and reabsorbed in the proximal tubule.
Kidney injury molecule-1 (KIM-1)	70–80 kDa	Cleaved and released into the lumen of the tubule. It facilitates repair of the damage by removing cellular debris and apoptotic bodies from the injured tubulointerstitial compartment.
N-acetyl-β-D glucosaminidase (NAG)	>130 kDa	Plasma NAG is not filtered through the glomeruli. It is released into the urine after renal tubule injury.
Liver-type fatty acid-binding protein (L-FABP)	14.2 kDa	Associated with structural and functional tubular damage. It is freely filtered and reabsorbed in the proximal tubule.
Megalin and Cubilin	Megalin 600 kDa Cubilin 460 kDa	Most proteins filtered through glomeruli have been identified as ligands of megalin, cubilin, or both. The central mechanism for protein reabsorption in the proximal tubule.
Alkaline phosphatase (ALP) and γ-glutamyltransferase (GGT)	ALP 70–120 kDa GGT 90 kDa	ALP originates from damaged renal tubules, and its levels are associated with the degree of damage. Increased GGT excretion in the urine reflects the damage of the brush-border membrane and the loss of microvilli.

Table 1. Principal functional and structural tubular biomarkers overexpressed in the urine and explored in clinical background of diabetic nephropathy [65–67].

cause albuminuria if proximal tubules are functioning normally and can reabsorb the excess albumin filtered from glomerulus. Other clinical study has also suggested the dissociation between albuminuria and increased glomerular leakage of albumin [70].

4.3. Predictive value in clinical studies

Studies using tubular biomarkers showed conflicting results regarding their predictive value for GFR decline or the development of albuminuria. In a retrospective analysis, two tubular injury biomarkers, $\beta2$ microglobulin and N-acetyl-β-D glucosaminidase (NAG), did not show prognostic utility for detecting GFR decline in type 2 DM (T2DM). However, histologic findings of interstitial fibrosis and tubular atrophy (IFTA) did have prognostic benefit. Both β2 microglobulin and NAG showed a statistically significant correlation with IFTA scores, identified as an independent predictor of progression to diabetic nephropathy [71]. In a nested case-control study from the diabetes control and complications trial (DCCT), both the baseline NAG and increase NAG over time predicted albuminuria independently [72]. A 3-year prospective study found that type 1 DM (T1DM) patients with high levels of urinary neutrophil gelatinase-associated lipocalin (NGAL) and kidney injury molecule-1 (KIM-1) had a rapid deterioration in GFR. This suggests that tubular injury is important for the progression of diabetic nephropathy [73]. Fu et al. [74] showed that NGAL increased significantly from healthy controls to normoalbuminuric, microalbuminuric, and macroalbuminuric patients with T2DM. Conway et al. [75] revealed that the uKIM-1/Cr ratio was elevated in T2DM patients with early-stage nephropathy, suggesting tubular injury. The uKIM-1/Cr ratio was correlated with a rapid decline in GFR and the severity of proteinuria. Soggiu et al. [76]showed that increased RBP4 and α1-microglobulin excretion could predict early-stage nephropathy in T1DM. In a retrospective cohort study of 1549 patients with T1DM, liver-type fatty acid-binding protein (L-FABP) was a valuable predictor of the progression of diabetic nephropathy, irrespective of disease stage [77]. Our laboratory reported that albuminuria is significantly correlated with three tubular biomarkers (KIM-1, NGAL, and L-FABP) during the early stage of diabetic nephropathy [78]. Our laboratory also reported results obtained from 237 patients with T2DM who were measured for NAP and cystatin C. Both biomarkers were significantly associated with the decline in eGFR after adjusting for clinical parameters [23]. Prospective studies are needed to confirm the clinical utility of tubular biomarkers in the early stage of diabetic nephropathy.

4.4. Proteomics and microRNA approach

Recently, many researches using high-throughput proteomics and microRNA (miRNA) approaches have been introduced in the field of diabetic nephropathy. These two novel approaches for discovering biomarkers can be used to explore diabetic nephropathy through multiple pathophysiological processes that can reflect complexed structural and functional pathways. Proteomics might provide dynamic profiles, reflecting the complexed pathophysiological changes that occur at different stages of diabetic nephropathy. Proteomics could serve as early biomarkers (e.g., CKD273 classifier, a panel consisting of 273 urinary peptides [79]) with a good predictive value in the clinical environments [80]. However, proteomic and miRNA approaches have yet not been able to replace albuminuria as a marker of diabetic nephropathy. miRNAs, which are small noncoding RNAs, are found in extracellular environment including various body fluids and function in posttranscriptional regulation of gene expression. The majority of miRNAs are located within the cell and can serve as a potential biomarker. In the urine, miRNAs are more stable in degradation than proteins and are valuable for urinary biomarkers. If miRNAs are handled and stored carefully, it could promote the discovery of novel urinary biomarkers for diabetic nephropathy. However, they were differentially expressed in T1DM and T2DM, and differed according to miRNA sources. In addition, miRNAs were reported to show gender-specific differences in T1DM [81]. Therefore, further studies are needed to optimize the utility of miRNAs in clinical practice.

5. Proximal tubules as therapeutic targets

Chronic hyperglycemia is an essential component of diabetes and the principal risk factor for microvascular complications, including diabetic nephropathy [82]. Patients with diabetes also have other risk factors such as obesity, systemic hypertension, and dyslipidemia. Despite advances in pharmacologic interventions (e.g., RAS blockers) to control these risk factors, the prevalence of diabetic nephropathy continues to rise and remains the leading cause of ESRD worldwide [83]. Several novel therapeutic strategies, including dual/triple RAS blockade and sulodexide and bardoxolone therapy, have been sought to improve renal outcome in diabetes [83]. However, these approaches proved either ineffective or harmful, suggesting that other strategies should be sought [84]. The optimal prevention and treatment of CKD in patients with diabetes requires the implementation of therapies that specifically consider the role played by proximal tubules [85]. The dimension and function of proximal tubules increase in response to a higher glucose load. These changes have been linked to an increase in GFR, or the so-called diabetic hyperfiltration [85]. Thus, considering the importance of proximal tubules in diabetic nephropathy, the development of novel antidiabetic agents, such as SGLT 2 inhibitors, could yield new tools to prevent diabetic nephropathy.

5.1. Glucose handling by the kidney

The glomeruli of normoglycemic healthy individuals filter ~140–160 g of glucose each day. This would result in a urinary loss of energy substrate equal to ~30% of the daily energy expenditure if not reclaimed by the renal tubules. Two glucose transporters are responsible for renal glucose reabsorption, SGLT1 and SGLT2, which are secondary active co-transporters located on the apical membrane that couple glucose reabsorption to sodium reabsorption. SGLT2 is located in the early (S1) proximal tubule and accounts for 90% of glucose reabsorption, while SGLT1 is located in the more distal part of the proximal tubule (S2/S3) and accounts for the remaining 10% [86].

5.2. Glucose reabsorption in the diabetic kidney

In diabetes, hyperglycemia is maintained by the alterations in kidney. Both renal gluconeogenesis and glucose reabsorption are increased in diabetic subjects [3]. Hyperglycemia increases the amount of glucose filtered through the kidney, and the maximum capacity of resorption for glucose is increased by ~30% to ~500–600 g/day in patients with type 2 diabetes [84]. If the filtered glucose load exceeds the threshold of proximal tubules in diabetes, glucosuria increases in a linear fashion. These latter changes occur in parallel with upregulated SGLT2 expression [87]. More specifically, an increased capacity for glucose transport may contribute to the enhanced renal glucose reabsorption seen in diabetes. Upregulated renal SGLT2 levels have been reported in both human cells and some animal models of type 1 and type 2 diabetes [88]. Proximal tubule growth (hypertrophy) is a key feature of early-stage diabetes, which may explain the increased capacity for renal glucose reabsorption [61]. However, it remains unclear whether SGLT2 upregulation is the result of proximal tubule hypertrophy in diabetes.

5.3. SGLT2 inhibition as a therapeutic target

Based on the observation that SGLT2 has an important role in renal glucose reabsorption, the proximal tubules of the kidney have been targeted to control the blood glucose. SGLT2 inhibitors are a novel class of antidiabetic drugs that recently entered the market. These medications target the kidney proximal tubules to block glucose reabsorption, thereby inducing urinary glucose excretion and reducing circulating plasma glucose levels. Their mechanisms of action are independent of the action of insulin and beta-cell function.

Phlorizin promotes glucosuria and lowers serum glucose levels in diabetic patients, and completely inhibits renal glucose reabsorption in humans [89]. However, the clinical use of phlorizin was not pursued due to poor intestinal absorption, low bioavailability, and lack of selectivity for SGLT2. Additionally, phlorizin is hydrolyzed to phloretin in the gut, which inhibits multiple GLUTs [90]. Thus, the development of SGLT2-specific inhibitor was an important breakthrough for therapies targeting renal glucose transport for blood glucose management [91].

Currently, the US Food and Drug Administration (FDA) and the European Medicines Agency (EMA) have approved three oral SGLT2 inhibitors (canagliflozin, dapagliflozin, and empagliflozin) for patients with type 2 diabetes. The SGLT2 inhibitors reduced HbA1C by 0.5–0.7% [92]. Additional drugs within this class are under development (**Table 2**). The glucose-lowering effect of SGLT2 inhibitors is closely related to the amount of filtered glucose. Since SGLT2 is responsible for >90% of glucose reabsorption by the kidney, its inhibition would be expected to induce a urinary glucose loss close to the filtered load (160–180 g/day in normoglycemia). However, SGLT2 inhibitor-associated urinary glucose excretion is only ~40–80 g/day in healthy individuals and patients with type 2 diabetes, suggesting that SGLT1

Generic name (trade name)	Company	Dosing	SGLT2/SGLT1 selectivity
Dapagliflozin (Forxiga/Farxiga)	AstraZeneca	5–10 mg QD	1400
Canagliflozin (Invokana)	Janssen	100–300 mg QD	160
Empagliflozin (Jardiance)	Boehringer Ingelheim	10–25 mg QD	5000
Ipragliflozin (Suglat)	Astellas Pharma	25–100 mg QD	570
Tofogliflozin (Apleway/Deberza)	Sanofi/Kowa	20 mg QD	1875
Luseogliflozin (Lusefi)	Taisho Pharmaceutical	2.5–5 mg QD	1770
Ertugliflozin (Steglatro)	Merck/Pfizer	1–25 mg QD	2200
Sotagliflozin[a] (N.A.)	Lexicon Pharmaceuticals	400 mg QD	20
Remogliflozin etabonate (N.A.)	BHV Pharma	100–400 mg QD	1100
Henagliflozin (N.A.)	Jiangsu HengRui Medicine	2.5–200 mg QD	1800

SGLT2/SGLT1, sodium-glucose cotransporter 2/sodium-glucose cotransporter 1; QD, once daily; N.A., not applicable.
[a]Dual SGLT1/2 inhibitor.

Table 2. SGLT2 inhibitors currently approved or in development.

has an important role in glucose reabsorption under SGLT2 inhibition [88]. SGLT2 inhibitor decreases insulin levels and increases glucagon levels. Thus, SGLT2 inhibitor enhances endogenous glucose production, thereby reducing the glucose-lowering efficacy [93].

5.3.1. Effects of SGLT2 inhibitors on renal and cardiovascular outcomes

The EMPA-REG OUTCOME and CANVAS trials investigated the effects of empagliflozin and canagliflozin on renal and cardiovascular outcomes in type 2 diabetes patient with high cardiovascular risk factors and an eGFR of $\geq$30 mL/min/1.73 m^2. In the EMPA-REG OUTCOME trial, empagliflozin was associated with a relative risk reduction of 39% in incident or worsening nephropathy (progression to macroalbuminuria, doubling of serum creatinine level, initiation of renal replacement therapy, or death from renal disease). Moreover, empagliflozin was associated with significant risk reductions of 44 and 55% in doubling serum creatinine and the initiation of renal replacement therapy, respectively [94]. Empagliflozin was also associated with relative risk reductions of 38, 35, and 32% in cardiovascular death, hospitalization for heart failure, and death from any cause, respectively. However, there was no risk reduction in nonfatal myocardial infarction or in nonfatal stroke [95]. In the CANVAS trial, canagliflozin was associated with relative risk reductions of 27 and 40% in the risk of albuminuria progression and composite renal outcome (40% reduction in eGFR, the need for renal replacement therapy, or death from renal cause), respectively [96]. Canagliflozin was also associated with a relative risk reduction of 14% in primary cardiovascular composite outcome (cardiovascular death, nonfatal myocardial infarction, or nonfatal stroke) [96].

5.3.2. SGLT2 inhibitors: beyond glucose lowering

The beneficial effects of SGLT2 inhibitors could be associated with a glucose-lowering effect. However, the small HbA1C reduction is unlikely to explain the rapid onset and effect size. Therefore, pleiotropic effects of SGLT2 inhibitor likely played a role (**Figure 3**). A meta-analysis of randomized controlled trial demonstrated that SGLT2 inhibitors decrease the systolic blood pressure by 3–6 mmHg in type 2 diabetes patients [92]. The blood pressure-lowering effect of SGLT2 inhibitors is partly associated with glycosuria-accompanied osmotic diuresis, which increases urine output by 200–600 mL/day. SGLT2 inhibitors also induce natriuresis by decreasing sodium reabsorption in the proximal tubules [84]. Additionally, a positive interaction between SGLTs and Na$^+$/H$^+$ exchanger-3 (NHE3), and the inhibition of NHE3 with phlorizin at sites associated with a reduced NHE3 activity have been described [97]. Since NHE3 in the early proximal tubule is responsible for up to 30% of fractional sodium reabsorption, its potentially downregulated activity on SGLT2 inhibition may contribute to natriuresis and subsequent GFR and blood pressure lowering; however, this hypothesis requires further study [98].

Clinical trials with SGLT2 inhibitors in patients with type 2 diabetes showed a significant weight reduction of ~1.7 kg or 2.4% compared with placebo [99]. While initial weight loss appears to result from SGLT2 inhibitor-associated osmotic diuresis, steady-state weight loss with SGLT2 inhibitor is thought to be associated with a reduction in body fat mass. In obese rat, SGLT2 inhibitor reduces fat mass with a steady calorie loss by increasing lipolysis and fatty acid oxidation. SGLT2 inhibitor-induced fat loss is also associated with the increased

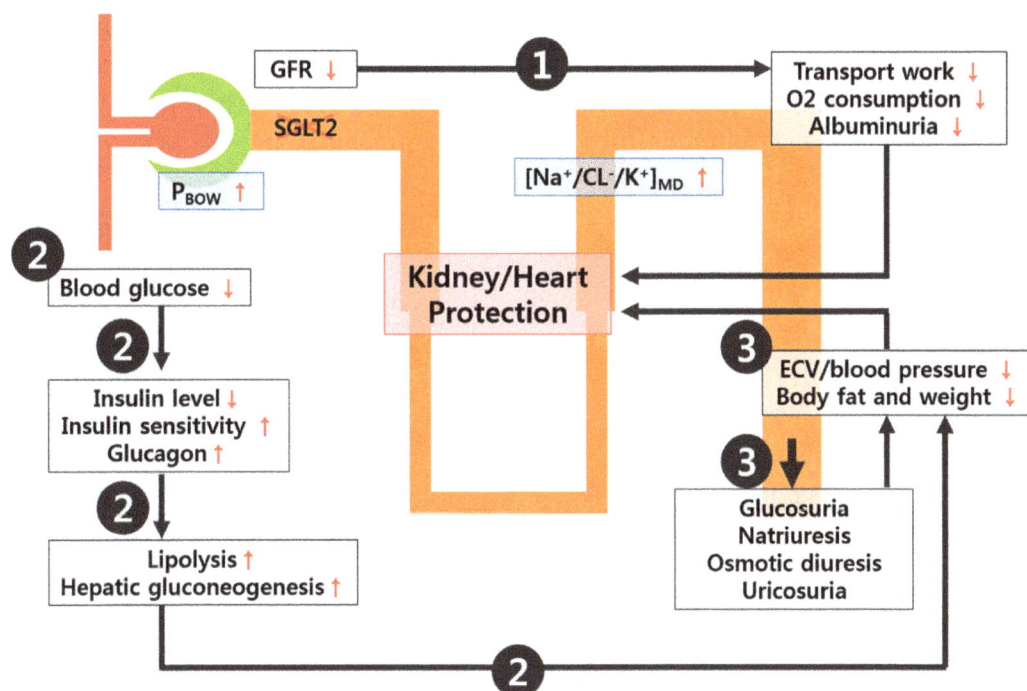

Figure 3. Pleiotropic effects of sodium-glucose cotransporter (SGLT2) inhibitor. SGLT2 inhibitor may have beneficial effects on kidney and heart via several pleiotropic mechanisms: (1) SGLT2 inhibitor blocks glucose hyper-reabsorption in the proximal tubule of the diabetic kidney, increasing the tubuloglomerular feedback signal at the macula densa ([Na$^+$/Cl$^-$/K$^+$]$_{MD}$) and hydrostatic pressure in Bowman's space (P$_{BOW}$). This reduces albuminuria and tubular transport work and, thus, renal oxygen consumption by decreasing glomerular hyperfiltration. (2) SGLT2 inhibition reduces insulin levels and increases insulin sensitivity and glucagon levels. As a consequence, lipolysis and hepatic gluconeogenesis are elevated. These metabolic adaptations reduce fat tissue and body weight. (3) SGLT2 inhibitors induce a modest osmotic diuresis, natriuresis, glucosuria, and uricosuria, which can reduce extracellular volume (ECV), blood pressure, serum uric acid levels, and body weight.

use of fatty acids instead of glucose as an energy source [100]. SGLT2 inhibitor has also been reported to reduce the body weight by reducing visceral and subcutaneous adipose tissue in type 2 diabetes patients [101].

Serum uric acid-lowering effect of SGLT2 inhibitor may be associated with the improved renal and cardiovascular outcome. SGLT2 inhibitor induces glycosuria, thereby facilitating intracellular uric acid exchange via GLUT9 isoform 2 at the proximal tubule, thereby enhancing urinary excretion of uric acid [102]. However, further study is mandatory to verify the precise mechanism of uricosuric effect of SGLT2 inhibitor.

Glomerular hyperfiltration is a detrimental process in diabetic nephropathy and increases intraglomerular pressure. The complicated interaction of hyperglycemia-induced structural and hemodynamic alterations causes the glomerular hyperfiltration [84]. By inducing baro-trauma and shear stress, it exacerbates albuminuria and likely contributes to the development and progression of CKD [84]. SGLT2 inhibition attenuates primary tubule hyper-reabsorption in diabetes and thereby reduces glomerular hyperfiltration. Specifically, SGLT2 inhibitors increase sodium delivery at the macula densa and subsequently activate tubuloglomerular feedback, which induce afferent arteriolar vasoconstriction and then reduce intraglomerular pressure [84]. Recent studies have also confirmed that the SGLT2 inhibitors lower GFR. The empagliflozin decreased the eGFR by 19% in type 1 diabetes patients. The canagliflozin also initially decreased GFR in patients with type 2 diabetes [103]. After an initial decrease in eGFR, canagliflozin-treated group showed the slower decline of eGFR compared with glimepiride-treated group over 2 years independently of glycemic effects [104].

5.3.3. SGLT2 inhibitors in diabetic CKD

Nephrons that survive in the advanced stages of CKD are assumed to hyper-filter as a way of compensating for the loss of other nephrons. In the short term, SGLT2 inhibitors decreased the eGFR in patients with type 2 diabetes and stage 2 or 3 CKD [105, 106]. In the long term, the amelioration of glomerular hyperfiltration by SGLT2 inhibitor in CKD may preserve the integrity of the remaining nephrons. This concept has also been suggested for angiotensin II inhibition. Indeed, both SGLT2 and angiotensin II inhibition confer additional renoprotective effect in type 2 diabetes patients with basal eGFR of >30 mL/min/1.73 m^2 [94].

5.4. SGLT2 inhibitors: future perspectives

The kidney and cardiovascular protection is likely to be attributed to the pleiotropic effects of SGLT2 (EMPA-REG OUTCOME and CANVAS trials). Future research is required to assess their ability to improve renal outcome in diabetic patients with more advanced CKD. The large trials with different SGLT2 inhibitors are ongoing to confirm whether their beneficial effects are drug-specific or represent a class effect. It is also important to investigate their effect in patients with nondiabetic kidney disease. In addition, dual SGLT1/2 inhibitors are under development to maximize the beneficial effect of SGLT2 inhibitors without causing side effects associated with SGLT1 inhibitors.

6. Conclusions

Although researchers are trying to determine the pathophysiology of diabetic nephropathy, our understanding remains incomplete. A recent paradigm shift to a tubulocentric concept for diabetic nephropathy implies that the proximal tubules have a central role in the disease process, rather than being secondarily affected by other components during the development of diabetic nephropathy. Representing a considerable step toward shifting the glomerulotubular balance, these new perspectives might lead to significant diagnostic and therapeutic advances in diabetic nephropathy.

Acknowledgements

This was supported by the Biomedical Research Institute Grant (Research Council, 2018; 2017B021 to J.H.K.) of the Pusan National University Hospital and the National Research Foundation of Korea (2018R1C1B6002854 to S.S.K., 2016R1A2B4008243 to S.H.S., 2017R1D1A1B03034926 to I.Y.K., and 2017R1C1B5016636 to S.M.L.).

Disclosures

The authors have nothing to disclose.

Author details

Sang Soo Kim[1,2]*, Jong Ho Kim[1,2], Su Mi Lee[4], Il Young Kim[1,3] and Sang Heon Song[1,2]

*Address all correspondence to: drsskim7@gmail.com

1 Department of Internal Medicine, Pusan National University School of Medicine, Yangsan, Gyeongsangnam-do, Republic of Korea

2 Biomedical Research Institute and Department of Internal Medicine, Pusan National University Hospital, Busan, Republic of Korea

3 Research Institute for Convergence of Biomedical Science and Technology and Department of Internal Medicine, Pusan National University Yangsan Hospital, Gyeongsangnam-do, Republic of Korea

4 Division of Nephrology, Department of Internal Medicine, Dong-A University Hospital, Busan, Korea

References

[1] Kim SS, Kim JH, Kim IJ. Current challenges in diabetic nephropathy: Early diagnosis and ways to improve outcomes. Endocrinology and Metabolism (Seoul, Korea). 2016;**31**:245-253. DOI: 10.3803/EnM.2016.31.2.245

[2] American Diabetes Association. Microvascular complications and foot care: Standards of medical care in diabetes-2018. Diabetes Care. 2018;**41**(Suppl 1):S105-S118. DOI: 10.2337/dc18-S010

[3] Tervaert TW, Mooyaart AL, Amann K, Cohen AH, Cook HT, Drachenberg CB, Ferrario F, Fogo AB, Haas M, de Heer E, Joh K, Noël LH, Radhakrishnan J, Seshan SV, Bajema IM, Bruijn JA, Renal Pathology Society. Pathologic classification of diabetic nephropathy. The Journal of the American Society of Nephrology. 2010;**21**:556-563. DOI: 10.1681/ASN.2010010010

[4] Alicic RZ, Rooney MT, Tuttle KR. Diabetic kidney disease: Challenges, progress, and possibilities. Clinical Journal of the American Society of Nephrology. 2017;**12**:2032-2045. DOI: 10.2215/CJN.11491116

[5] Eknoyan G, Nagy J. A history of diabetes mellitus or how a disease of the kidneys evolved into a kidney disease. Advances in Chronic Kidney Disease. 2005;**12**:223-229

[6] Mogensen CE, Christensen CK, Vittinghus E. The stages in diabetic renal disease. With emphasis on the stage of incipient diabetic nephropathy. Diabetes. 1983;**32**(Suppl 2):64-78

[7] Kasper D, Fauci A, Hauser S, Longo D, Jameson JL, Loscalzo J. Harrison's Principles of Internal Medicine. 19th ed. New York: McGraw Hill Education Medical; 2015. p. 2425

[8] Pugliese G. Updating the natural history of diabetic nephropathy. Acta Diabetologica. 2014;**51**:905-915. DOI: 10.1007/s00592-014-0650-7

[9] Araki S, Haneda M, Sugimoto T, Isono M, Isshiki K, Kashiwagi A, Koya D. Factors associated with frequent remission of microalbuminuria in patients with type 2 diabetes. Diabetes. 2005;**54**:2983-2987

[10] Tuttle KR, Bakris GL, Bilous RW, Chiang JL, de Boer IH, Goldstein-Fuchs J, Hirsch IB, Kalantar-Zadeh K, Narva AS, Navaneethan SD, Neumiller JJ, Patel UD, Ratner RE, Whaley-Connell AT, Molitch ME. Diabetic kidney disease: A report from an ADA consensus conference. Diabetes Care. Oct 2014;**37**(10):2864-2883. DOI: 10.2337/dc14-1296

[11] Babazono T, Nyumura I, Toya K, Hayashi T, Ohta M, Suzuki K, Kiuchi Y, Iwamoto Y. Higher levels of urinary albumin excretion within the normal range predict faster decline in glomerular filtration rate in diabetic patients. Diabetes Care. 2009;**32**:1518-1520. DOI: 10.2337/dc08-2151

[12] Gerstein HC, Mann JF, Yi Q, Zinman B, Dinneen SF, Hoogwerf B, Hallé JP, Young J, Rashkow A, Joyce C, Nawaz S, Yusuf S, HOPE Study Investigators. Albuminuria and risk of cardiovascular events, death, and heart failure in diabetic and nondiabetic individuals. Journal of the American Medical Association. 2001;**286**:421-426

[13] Bilous R. Microvascular disease: What does the UKPDS tell us about diabetic nephropathy? Diabetic Medicine. 2008;**25**:25-29. DOI: 10.1111/j.1464-5491.2008.02496.x

[14] Perkins BA, Ficociello LH, Silva KH, Finkelstein DM, Warram JH, Krolewski AS. Regression of microalbuminuria in type 1 diabetes. The New England Journal of Medicine. 2003;**348**:2285-2293

[15] Vaidya VS, Niewczas MA, Ficociello LH, Johnson AC, Collings FB, Warram JH, Krolewski AS, Bonventre JV. Regression of microalbuminuria in type 1 diabetes is associated with lower levels of urinary tubular injury biomarkers, kidney injury molecule-1, and N-acetyl-β-D-glucosaminidase. Kidney International. 2011;**79**:464-470. DOI: 10.1038/ki.2010.404

[16] Atta MG, Baptiste-Roberts K, Brancati FL, Gary TL. The natural course of microalbuminuria among African Americans with type 2 diabetes: A 3-year study. The American Journal of Medicine. 2009;**122**:62-72. DOI: 10.1016/j.amjmed.2008.07.023

[17] Jansson FJ, Forsblom C, Harjutsalo V, Thorn LM, Wadén J, Elonen N, Ahola AJ, Saraheimo M, Groop PH, FinnDiane Study Group. Regression of albuminuria and its association with incident cardiovascular outcomes and mortality in type 1 diabetes: The FinnDiane study. Diabetologia. 2018;**61**:1203-1211. DOI: 10.1007/s00125-018-4564-8

[18] Araki S, Haneda M, Koya D, Hidaka H, Sugimoto T, Isono M, Isshiki K, Chin-Kanasaki M, Uzu T, Kashiwagi A. Reduction in microalbuminuria as an integrated indicator

for renal and cardiovascular risk reduction in patients with type 2 diabetes. Diabetes. 2007;**56**:1727-1730

[19] Ibsen H, Olsen MH, Wachtell K, Borch-Johnsen K, Lindholm LH, Mogensen CE, Dahlöf B, Devereux RB, de Faire U, Fyhrquist F, Julius S, Kjeldsen SE, Lederballe-Pedersen O, Nieminen MS, Omvik P, Oparil S, Wan Y. Reduction in albuminuria translates to reduction in cardiovascular events in hypertensive patients: Losartan intervention for endpoint reduction in hypertension study. Hypertension. 2005;**45**:198-202

[20] Carrol MF, Temte JL. Proteinuria in adult: A diagnostic approach. American Family Physician. 2000;**62**:1333-1340

[21] Katayev A, Zebelman AM, Sharp TM, Flynn S, Bernstein RK. Prevalence of isolated non-albumin proteinuria in the US population tested for both, urine total protein and urine albumin: An unexpected discovery. Clinical Biochemistry. 2017;**50**:262-269. DOI: 10.1016/j.clinbiochem.2016.11.030

[22] Ballantyne FC, Gibbons J, O'Reilly DS. Urine albumin should replace total protein for the assessment of glomerular proteinuria. Annals of Clinical Biochemistry. 1993;**30**(1):101-103

[23] Kim SS, Song SH, Kim IJ, Jeon YK, Kim BH, Kwak IS, Lee EK, Kim YK. Urinary cystatin C and tubular proteinuria predict progression of diabetic nephropathy. Diabetes Care. 2013;**36**:656-661

[24] Kim SS, Song SH, Kim IJ, Kim WJ, Jeon YK, Kim BH, Kwak IS, Lee EK, Kim YK. Nonalbuminuric proteinuria as a biomarker for tubular damage in early development of nephropathy with type 2 diabetic patients. Diabetes/Metabolism Research and Reviews. 2014;**30**:736-741. DOI: 10.2337/dc12-0849

[25] Kim JH, Kim SS, Kim IJ, Lee MJ, Jeon YK, Kim BH, Song SH, Kim YK. Nonalbumin proteinuria is a simple and practical predictor of the progression of early-stage type 2 diabetic nephropathy. Journal of Diabetes and its Complications. 2017;**31**:395-399. DOI: 10.1016/j.jdiacomp.2016

[26] Chen C, Wang C, Hu C, Han Y, Zhao L, Zhu X, Xiao L, Sun L. Normoalbuminuric diabetic kidney disease. Frontiers in Medicine. 2017;**11**:310-318. DOI: 10.1007/s11684-017-0542-7

[27] Retnakaran R, Cull CA, Thorne KI, Adler AI, Holman RR, UKPDS Study Group. Risk factors for renal dysfunction in type 2 diabetes: U.K. prospective diabetes study 74. Diabetes. 2006;**55**:1832-1839

[28] An JH, Cho YM, Yu HG, Jang HC, Park KS, Kim SY, Lee HK. The clinical characteristics of normoalbuminuric renal insufficiency in Korean type 2 diabetic patients: A possible early stage renal complication. Journal of Korean Medical Science. 2009;**24**:S75-S81. DOI: 10.3346/jkms.2009.24.S1.S75

[29] Ekinci EI, Jerums G, Skene A, Crammer P, Power D, Cheong KY, Panagiotopoulos S, McNeil K, Baker ST, Fioretto P, Macisaac RJ. Renal structure in normoalbuminuric and albuminuric patients with type 2 diabetes and impaired renal function. Diabetes Care. 2013;**36**:3620-3626. DOI: 10.2337/dc12-2572

[30] Yu SM, Bonventre JV. Acute kidney injury and progression of diabetic kidney disease. Advances in Chronic Kidney Disease. 2018;**25**:166-180. DOI: 10.1053/j.ackd.2017.12.005

[31] Najafian B, Kim Y, Crosson JT, Mauer M. Atubular glomeruli and glomerulotubular junction abnormalities in diabetic nephropathy. The Journal of the American Society of Nephrology. 2003;**14**:908-917

[32] Krolewski AS. Progressive renal decline: The new paradigm of diabetic nephropathy in type 1 diabetes. Diabetes Care. 2015;**38**:954-962. DOI: 10.2337/dc15-0184

[33] Looker HC, Colombo M, Hess S, Brosnan MJ, Farran B, Dalton RN, Wong MC, Turner C, Palmer CN, Nogoceke E, Groop L, Salomaa V, Dunger DB, Agakov F, McKeigue PM, Colhoun HM, Investigators SUMMIT. Biomarkers of rapid chronic kidney disease progression in type 2 diabetes. Kidney International. Oct 2015;**88**(4):888-896. DOI: 10.1038/ki.2015.199

[34] Nowak N, Skupien J, Smiles AM, Yamanouchi M, Niewczas MA, Galecki AT, Duffin KL, Breyer MD, Pullen N, Bonventre JV, Krolewski AS. Markers of early progressive renal decline in type 2 diabetes suggest different implications for etiological studies and prognostic tests development. Kidney International. Feb 2, 2018 [Epub ahead of print]. DOI: 10.1016/j.kint.2017.11.024

[35] Kimmelstiel P, Wilson C. Intercapillary lesions in the glomeruli of the kidney. The American Journal of Pathology. 1936;**12**:83-98.7

[36] Gnudi L. Cellular and molecular mechanisms of diabetic glomerulopathy. Nephrology, Dialysis, Transplantation. 2012;**27**:2642-2649. DOI: 10.1093/ndt/gfs121

[37] Gilbert RE. Proximal tubulopathy: Prime mover and key therapeutic target in diabetic kidney disease. Diabetes. 2017;**66**:791-800. DOI: 10.2337/db16-0796

[38] Gilbert RE, Cooper ME. The tubulointerstitium in progressive diabetic kidney disease: More than an aftermath of glomerular injury? Kidney International. 1999;**56**:1627-1637

[39] Marcussen N. Atubular glomeruli and the structural basis for chronic renal failure. Laboratory Investigation. 1992;**66**:265-284

[40] Marcussen N. Tubulointerstitial damage leads to atubular glomeruli: Significance and possible role in progression. Nephrology, Dialysis, Transplantation. 2000;**15**:74-75

[41] White KE, Marshall SM, Bilous RW. Prevalence of atubular glomeruli in type 2 diabetic patients with nephropathy. Nephrology, Dialysis, Transplantation. 2008;**23**:3539-3545. DOI: 10.1093/ndt/gfn351

[42] Hasegawa K, Wakino S, Simic P, Sakamaki Y, Minakuchi H, Fujimura K, Hosoya K, Komatsu M, Kaneko Y, Kanda T, Kubota E, Tokuyama H, Hayashi K, Guarente L, Itoh H. Renal tubular Sirt1 attenuates diabetic albuminuria by epigenetically suppressing Claudin-1 overexpression in podocytes. Nature Medicine. 2013;**19**:1496-1504. DOI: 10.1038/nm.3363

[43] Nihalani D, Susztak K. Sirt1-Claudin-1 crosstalk regulates renal function. Nature Medicine. 2013;**19**:1371-1372. DOI: 10.1038/nm.3386

[44] Grgic I, Campanholle G, Bijol V, Wang C, Sabbisetti VS, Ichimura T, Humphreys BD, Bonventre JV. Targeted proximal tubule injury triggers interstitial fibrosis and glomerulosclerosis. Kidney International. 2012;**82**:172-183. DOI: 10.1038/ki.2012.20

[45] Yu Y, Jin H, Holder D, Ozer JS, Villarreal S, Shughrue P, Shi S, Figueroa DJ, Clouse H, Su M, Muniappa N, Troth SP, Bailey W, Seng J, Aslamkhan AG, Thudium D, Sistare FD, Gerhold DL. Urinary biomarkers trefoil factor 3 and albumin enable early detection of kidney tubular injury. Nature Biotechnology. 2010;**28**:470-477. DOI: 10.1038/nbt.1624

[46] Bonventre JV. Can we target tubular damage to prevent renal function decline in diabetes? Seminars in Nephrology. 2012;**32**:452-462. DOI: 10.1016/j.semnephrol.2012.07.008

[47] Körner A, Eklöf AC, Celsi G, Aperia A. Increased renal metabolism in diabetes. Mechanism and functional implications. Diabetes. 1994;**43**:629-633

[48] Chang YK, Choi H, Jeong JY, Na KR, Lee KW, Lim BJ, Choi DE. Dapagliflozin, SGLT2 inhibitor, attenuates renal ischemia-reperfusion injury. PLoS One. 2016;**11**:e0158810. DOI: 10.1371/journal.pone.0158810

[49] Alsahli M, Gerich JE. Renal glucose metabolism in normal physiological conditions and in diabetes. Diabetes Research and Clinical Practice. Nov 2017;**133**:1-9. DOI: 10.1016/j.diabres.2017.07.033

[50] Khan S, Cleveland RP, Koch CJ, Schelling JR. Hypoxia induces renal tubular epithelial cell apoptosis in chronic renal disease. Laboratory Investigation. 1999;**79**:1089-1099

[51] Khan S, Koepke A, Jarad G, Schlessman K, Cleveland RP, Wang B, Konieczkowski M, Schelling JR. Apoptosis and JNK activation are differentially regulated by Fas expression level in renal tubular epithelial cells. Kidney International. 2001;**60**:65-76

[52] Orphanides C, Fine LG, Norman JT. Hypoxia stimulates proximal tubular cell matrix production via a TGF-beta1-independent mechanism. Kidney International. 1997;**52**:637-647

[53] Fine LG, Norman JT. Chronic hypoxia as a mechanism of progression of chronic kidney diseases: From hypothesis to novel therapeutics. Kidney International. 2008;**74**:867-872. DOI: 10.1038/ki.2008.350

[54] Kim SS, Shin N, Bae SS, Lee MY, Rhee H, Kim IY, Seong EY, Lee DW, Lee SB, Kwak IS, Lovett DH, Song SH. Enhanced expression of two discrete isoforms of matrix metalloproteinase-2 in experimental and human diabetic nephropathy. PLoS One. 2017;**12**:e0171625. DOI: 10.1371/journal.pone.0171625

[55] Ceron CS, Baligand C, Joshi S, Wanga S, Cowley PM, Walker JP, Song SH, Mahimkar R, Baker AJ, Raffai RL, Wang ZJ, Lovett DH. An intracellular matrix metalloproteinase-2 isoform induces tubular regulated necrosis: Implications for acute kidney injury. American Journal of Physiology. Renal Physiology. 2017;**312**. DOI: F1166-F1183. DOI: 10.1152/ajprenal.00461

[56] Thomas MC, Burns WC, Cooper ME. Tubular changes in early diabetic nephropathy. Advances in Chronic Kidney Disease. 2005;**12**:177-186

[57] Thakar CV, Christianson A, Himmelfarb J, Leonard AC. Acute kidney injury episodes and chronic kidney disease risk in diabetes mellitus. Clinical Journal of the American Society of Nephrology. 2011;6:2567-2572. DOI: 10.2215/CJN.01120211

[58] Monseu M, Gand E, Saulnier PJ, Ragot S, Piguel X, Zaoui P, Rigalleau V, Marechaud R, Roussel R, Hadjadj S, Halimi JM, SURDIAGENE Study Group. Acute kidney injury predicts major adverse outcomes in diabetes: Synergic impact with low glomerular filtration rate and albuminuria. Diabetes Care. 2015;38:2333-2340. DOI: 10.2337/dc15-1222

[59] Comper WD, Haraldsson B, Deen WM. Resolved: Normal glomeruli filter nephrotic levels of albumin. The Journal of the American Society of Nephrology. 2008;19:427-432. DOI: 10.1681/ASN.2007090997

[60] Russo LM, Sandoval RM, Campos SB, Molitoris BA, Comper WD, Brown D. Impaired tubular uptake explains albuminuria in early diabetic nephropathy. The Journal of the American Society of Nephrology. 2009;20:489-494. DOI: 10.1681/ASN.2008050503

[61] Zeni L, Norden AGW, Cancarini G, Unwin RJ. A more tubulocentric view of diabetic kidney disease. Journal of Nephrology. 2017;30:701-717. DOI: 10.1007/s40620-017-0423-9

[62] Norden AG, Lapsley M, Lee PJ, Pusey CD, Scheinman SJ, Tam FW, Thakker RV, Unwin RJ, Wrong O. Glomerular protein sieving and implications for renal failure in Fanconi syndrome. Kidney International. 2001;60:1885-1892

[63] Dickson LE, Wagner MC, Sandoval RM, Molitoris BA. The proximal tubule and albuminuria: Really! The Journal of the American Society of Nephrology. 2014;25:443-453. DOI: 10.1681/ASN.2013090950

[64] Viazzi F, Cappadona F, Pontremoli R. Microalbuminuria in primary hypertension: A guide to optimal patient management? Journal of Nephrology. 2016;29(6):747-753. DOI: 10.1016/j.jdiacomp.2016.10.030

[65] Gluhovschi C, Gluhovschi G, Petrica L, Timar R, Velciov S, Ionita I, Kaycsa A, Timar B. Urinary biomarkers in the assessment of early diabetic nephropathy. Journal of Diabetes Research. 2016;2016:4626125. DOI: 10.1371/journal.pone.0112538

[66] Moresco RN, Sangoi MB, De Carvalho JA, Tatsch E, Bochi GV. Diabetic nephropathy: Traditional to proteomic markers. Clinica chimica acta. International Journal of Clinical Chemistry. 2013;421:17-30. DOI: 10.1016/j.cca.2013.02.019

[67] Burling KA, Cutillas PR, Church D, Lapsley M, Norden AG. Analysis of molecular forms of urine retinol-binding protein in Fanconi syndrome and design of an accurate immunoassay. Clinica chimica acta. International Journal of Clinical Chemistry. 2012;413(3-4):483-489. DOI: 10.1016/j.cca.2011.11.007

[68] Bernard A, Amor AO, Viau C, Lauwerys R. The renal uptake of proteins: A nonselective process in conscious rats. Kidney International. 1988;34(2):175-185

[69] Norden AG, Scheinman SJ, Deschodt-Lanckman MM, Lapsley M, Nortier JL, Thakker RV, Unwin RJ, Wrong O. Tubular proteinuria defined by a study of Dent's (CLCN5 mutation) and other tubular diseases. Kidney International. 2000;57(1):240-249. DOI: 10.1046/j.1523-1755.2000.00847.x

[70] Petrica L, Vlad A, Gluhovschi G, Gadalean F, Dumitrascu V, Gluhovschi C, Velciov S, Bob F, Vlad D, Popescu R, Milas O, Ursoniu S. Proximal tubule dysfunction is associated with podocyte damage biomarkers nephrin and vascular endothelial growth factor in type 2 diabetes mellitus patients: A crosssectional study. PLoS One. 2014;9(11):e112538. DOI: 10.1371/journal.pone.0112538

[71] Mise K, Hoshino J, Ueno T, Hazue R, Hasegawa J, Sekine A, Sumida K, Hiramatsu R, Hasegawa E, Yamanouchi M, Hayami N, Suwabe T, Sawa N, Fujii T, Hara S, Ohashi K, Takaichi K, Ubara Y. Prognostic value of tubulo-interstitial lesions, urinary N-acetyl-beta-d-glucosaminidase, and urinary beta2-microglobulin in patients with type 2 diabetes and biopsy-proven diabetic nephropathy. The Clinical Journal of the American Society of Nephrology. 2016;11(4):593-601. DOI: 10.2215/CJN.04980515

[72] Kern EF, Erhard P, Sun W, Genuth S, Weiss MF. Early urinary markers of diabetic kidney disease: A nested case-control study from the diabetes control and complications trial (DCCT). The American Journal of Kidney Diseases (AJKD): Official Journal of the National KidneyFoundation. 2010;55(5):824-834. DOI: 10.1053/j.ajkd.2009.11.009

[73] Nielsen SE, Andersen S, Zdunek D, Hess G, Parving HH, Rossing P. Tubular markers do not predict the decline in glomerular filtration rate in type 1 diabetic patients with overt nephropathy. Kidney International. 2011;79(10):1113-1118. DOI: 10.1038/ki.2010.554

[74] Fu WJ, Xiong SL, Fang YG, Wen S, Chen ML, Deng RT, Zheng L, Wang SB, Pen LF, Wang Q. Urinary tubular biomarkers in short-term type 2 diabetes mellitus patients: A cross-sectional study. Journal of Endocrinology. 2012;41(1):82-88. DOI: 10.1007/s12020-011-9509-7

[75] Conway BR, Manoharan D, Manoharan D, Jenks S, Dear JW, McLachlan S, Strachan MW, Price JF. Measuring urinary tubular biomarkers in type 2 diabetes does not add prognostic value beyond established risk factors. Kidney International. 2012;82(7):812-818. DOI: 10.1038/ki.2012.218

[76] Soggiu A, Piras C, Bonizzi L, Hussein HA, Pisanu S, Roncada P. A discovery-phase urine proteomics investigation in type 1 diabetes. Acta Diabetologica. 2012;49(6):453-464. DOI: 10.1007/s00592-012-0407-0

[77] Panduru NM, Forsblom C, Saraheimo M, Thorn L, Bierhaus A, Humpert PM, Groop PH, FinnDiane Study G. Urinary liver-type fatty acid-binding protein and progression of diabetic nephropathy in type 1 diabetes. Diabetes Care. 2013;36(7):2077-2083. DOI: 10.2337/dc12-1868

[78] Kim SS, Song SH, Kim IJ, Yang JY, Lee JG, Kwak IS, Kim YK. Clinical implication of urinary tubular markers in the early stage of nephropathy with type 2 diabetic patients. Diabetes Research and Clinical Practice. 2012;97(2):251-257. DOI: 10.1016/j.diabres.2012.02.019

[79] Zurbig P, Jerums G, Hovind P, Macisaac RJ, Mischak H, Nielsen SE, Panagiotopoulos S, Persson F, Rossing P. Urinary proteomics for early diagnosis in diabetic nephropathy. Diabetes. 2012;61(12):3304-3313. DOI: 10.2337/db12-0348

[80] Papale M, Di Paolo S, Vocino G, Rocchetti MT, Gesualdo L. Proteomics and diabetic nephropathy: What have we learned from a decade of clinical proteomics studies? Journal of Nephrology. 2014;27:221-228. DOI: 10.1007/s40620-014-0044-5

[81] Argyropoulos C, Wang K, Bernardo J, Ellis D, Orchard T, Galas D, Johnson JP. Urinary MicroRNA profiling predicts the development of microalbuminuria in patients with type 1 diabetes. Journal of Clinical Medicine. 2015;**4**(7):1498-1517. DOI: 10.3390/jcm4071498

[82] Muskiet MH, Tonneijck L, Smits MM, Kramer MH, Heerspink HJ, van Raalte DH. Pleiotropic effects of type 2 diabetes management strategies on renal risk factors. The Lancet Diabetes and Endocrinology. 2015;**3**:367-381. DOI: 10.1016/S2213-8587(15)00030-3

[83] Atkins RC, Zimmet P. Diabetic kidney disease: Act now or pay later. Kidney International. 2010;**77**:375-377. DOI: 10.1038/ki.2009.509

[84] Bommel EJ, Muskiet MH, Tonneijck L, Kramer MH, Nieuwdorp M, van Raalte DH. SGLT2 inhibition in the diabetic kidney-from mechanisms to clinical outcome. Clinical Journal of the American Society of Nephrology. 2017;**12**:700-710. DOI: 10.2215/CJN.06080616

[85] Thomson SC, Vallon V, Blantz RC. Kidney function in early diabetes: The tubular hypothesis of glomerular filtration. American Journal of Physiology. Renal Physiology. 2004;**286**:F8-F15

[86] Rieg T, Masuda T, Gerasimova M, Mayoux E, Platt K, Powell DR, et al. Increase in SGLT1-mediated transport explains renal glucose reabsorption during genetic and pharmacological SGLT2 inhibition in euglycemia. American Journal of Physiology. Renal Physiology. 2014;**306**:F188-F193. DOI: 10.1152/ajprenal.00518.2013

[87] Rahmoune H, Thompson PW, Ward JM, Smith CD, Hong G, Brown J. Glucose transporters in human renal proximal tubular cells isolated from the urine of patients with non-insulin-dependent diabetes. Diabetes. 2005;**54**:3427-3434

[88] Vallon V. The mechanisms and therapeutic potential of SGLT2 inhibitors in diabetes mellitus. Annual Review of Medicine. 2015;**66**:255-270. DOI: 10.1146/annurev-med-051013-110046

[89] Chasis H, Jolliffe N, Smith HW. The action of phlorizin on the excretion of glucose, xylose, sucrose, creatinine and urea by man. The Journal of Clinical Investigation. 1933;**12**:1083-1090

[90] Chao EC, Henry RR. SGLT2 inhibition – A novel strategy for diabetes treatment. Nature Reviews. Drug Discovery. 2010;**9**:551-559. DOI: 10.1038/nrd3180

[91] Vallon V, Thomson SC. Targeting renal glucose reabsorption to treat hyperglycaemia: The pleiotropic effects of SGLT2 inhibition. Diabetologia. 2017;**60**:215-225. DOI: 10.1007/s00125-016-4157-3

[92] Monami M, Nardini C, Mannucci E. Efficacy and safety of sodium glucose co-transport-2 inhibitors in type 2 diabetes: A meta-analysis of randomized clinical trials. Diabetes, Obesity and Metabolism. 2014;**16**:457-466. DOI: 10.1111/dom

[93] Cefalu WT. Paradoxical insights into whole body metabolic adaptations following SGLT2 inhibition. The Journal of Clinical Investigation. 2014;**124**:485-487. DOI: 10.1172/JCI74297

[94] Wanner C, Inzucchi SE, Lachin JM, Fitchett D, von Eynatten M, Mattheus M, et al. Empagliflozin and progression of kidney disease in type 2 diabetes. The New England Journal of Medicine. 2016;**375**:323-334. DOI: 10.1056/NEJMoa1515920

[95] Zinman B, Wanner C, Lachin JM, Fitchett D, Bluhmki E, Hantel S, et al. Empagliflozin, cardiovascular outcomes, and mortality in type 2 diabetes. The New England Journal of Medicine. 2015;**373**:2117-2128. DOI: 10.1056/NEJMoa1504720

[96] Neal B, Perkovic V, Mahaffey KW, de Zeeuw D, Fulcher G, Erondu N, et al. Canagliflozin and cardiovascular and renal events in type 2 diabetes. The New England Journal of Medicine. 2017;**377**:644-657. DOI: 10.1056/NEJMoa1611925

[97] Pessoa TD, Campos LC, Carraro-Lacroix L, Girardi AC, Malnic G. Functional role of glucose metabolism, osmotic stress, and sodium-glucose cotransporter isoform-mediated transport on Na^+/H^+ exchanger isoform 3 activity in the renal proximal tubule. The Journal of the American Society of Nephrology. 2014;**25**:2028-2039. DOI: 10.1681/ASN.2013060588

[98] Gallo LA, Wright EM, Vallon V. Probing SGLT2 as a therapeutic target for diabetes: Basic physiology and consequences. Diabetes and Vascular Disease Research. 2015;**12**:78-89. DOI: 10.1177/1479164114561992

[99] Vasilakou D, Karagiannis T, Athanasiadou E, Mainou M, Liakos A, Bekiari E, et al. Sodium-glucose cotransporter 2 inhibitors for type 2 diabetes: A systematic review and meta-analysis. Annals of Internal Medicine. 2013;**159**:262-274. DOI: 10.7326/0003-4819-159-4-201308200-00007

[100] Yokono M, Takasu T, Hayashizaki Y, Mitsuoka K, Kihara R, Muramatsu Y, et al. SGLT2 selective inhibitor ipragliflozin reduces body fat mass by increasing fatty acid oxidation in high-fat diet-induced obese rats. European Journal of Pharmacology. 2014;**727**:66-74. DOI: 10.1016/j.ejphar.2014.01.040

[101] Bolinder J, Ljunggren O, Kullberg J, Johansson L, Wilding J, Langkilde AM, et al. Effects of dapagliflozin on body weight, total fat mass, and regional adipose tissue distribution in patients with type 2 diabetes mellitus with inadequate glycemic control on metformin. The Journal of Clinical Endocrinology and Metabolism. 2012;**97**:1020-1031. DOI: 10.1210/jc.2016-3284

[102] Chino Y, Samukawa Y, Sakai S, Nakai Y, Yamaguchi J, Nakanishi T, et al. SGLT2 inhibitor lowers serum uric acid through alteration of uric acid transport activity in renal tubule by increased glycosuria. Biopharmaceutics and Drug Disposition. 2014;**35**:391-404. DOI: 10.1002/bdd.1909

[103] Cherney DZ, Perkins BA, Soleymanlou N, Maione M, Lai V, Lee A, et al. Renal hemodynamic effect of sodium-glucose cotransporter 2 inhibition in patients with type 1 diabetes mellitus. Circulation. 2014;**129**:587-597. DOI: 10.1161/CIRCULATIONAHA.113.005081

[104] Heerspink HJ, Desai M, Jardine M, Balis D, Meininger G, Perkovic V. Canagliflozin slows progression of renal function decline independently of glycemic effects. The Journal of the American Society of Nephrology. 2017;**28**:368-375. DOI: 10.1681/ASN.2016030278

[105] Yale JF, Bakris G, Cariou B, Yue D, David-Neto E, Xi L, et al. Efficacy and safety of canagliflozin in subjects with type 2 diabetes and chronic kidney disease. Diabetes, Obesity and Metabolism. 2013;**15**:463-473. DOI: 10.1111/dom.12090

[106] Barnett AH, Mithal A, Manassie J, Jones R, Rattunde H, Woerle HJ, et al. Efficacy and safety of empagliflozin added to existing antidiabetes treatment in patients with type 2 diabetes and chronic kidney disease: A randomised, double-blind, placebo-controlled trial. The Lancet Diabetes and Endocrinology. 2014;**2**:369-384. DOI: 10.1016/S2213-8587(13)70208-0

3

C3 Glomerulopathy

Nika Kojc

Abstract

Understanding the role of alternative complement pathway dysregulation in membranoproliferative glomerulonephritis (MPGN) has led to a new classification into two subgroups: immune complex-mediated MPGN and complement-mediated MPGN. Immune complex-mediated MPGN results from the deposition of immunoglobulin deposits and complements component C3 driven by classical complement pathway activation, while complement-mediated disease may be associated with complement alternative pathway dysregulation and is a new entity, C3 glomerulopathy. C3 glomerulopathy is an umbrella term, encompassing dense deposit disease (DDD), former MPGN type II, and C3 glomerulonephritis. C3 glomerulonephritis comprises examples of MPGN types I and III, in which immunofluorescence reveals predominant C3 deposits. By light microscopy, distinctive histologic patterns can be observed in both entities, including membranoproliferative, mesangial proliferative, crescentic and acute proliferative and exudative patterns, of which the membranoproliferative pattern seems to be the most common. DDD is defined by the presence of dense osmiophilic transformation of the glomerular basement membrane (GBM) on electron microscopy (EM). Only EM enables definite distinction of DDD from C3 glomerulonephritis. C3 glomerulopathy is a heterogeneous disease; genetic or acquired complement alternative pathway abnormalities have been identified in up to 40% of patients, including mutations in complement factors or autoantibodies directed against them.

Keywords: C3 glomerulopathy, C3 glomerulonephritis, dense deposit disease, membranoproliferative glomerulonephritis, complement alternative pathway dysregulation, complement regulation, CFHR5 nephropathy, C3 nephritic factor, eculizumab

1. Introduction

C3 glomerulopathy is a recently defined glomerular disease, characterized by predominant C3 complement component (C3) deposits in the glomeruli in the absence of a significant amount of immunoglobulin and without deposition of C1q and C4. The accumulation of C3 without a significant amount of classical or lectin complement component in the glomeruli suggests dysregulation of the alternative complement pathway as the underlying pathogenetic mechanism.

Glomerular C3 deposits confirmed by immunohistochemistry correspond to electron dense deposits seen on electron microscopy (EM). By light microscopy, distinctive histologic patterns can be observed, including membranoproliferative, mesangial proliferative, crescentic and acute proliferative and exudative patterns, of which the membranoproliferative pattern seems to be the most common [1–3]. The recognition of C3 glomerulopathy led to a major revision of the understanding of the entity of membranoproliferative glomerulonephritis (MPGN) [1, 4, 5].

2. Historical overview of membranoproliferative glomerulonephritis

Rather than a disease, MPGN is a morphologic pattern of glomerular injury, characterized on light microscopy by mesangial hypercellularity and thickening of the capillary walls, resulting in glomerular capillary wall remodeling. In the active phase, a proliferative and exudative pattern predominates, whereas in the reparative phase, mesangial expansion occurs, together with double contour formation and mesangial interposition seen on EM [6, 7].

Without knowledge of the pathogenesis, MPGN was traditionally classified based on histologic features defined by light microscopy and the location of the deposits as observed by EM. Three types of MPGN were recognized: MPGN types I, II and III [7–9].

MPGN type I was characterized by mesangial and subendothelial deposits, with marked mesangial interposition and double contour formation (**Figure 1**) [9]. Type III, defined by mesangial, subendothelial and subepithelial deposits, was further subdivided into two variants: the Burkholder variant and Anders-Strife variant, describing different patterns of electron dense deposits and disorganization of the glomerular basement membrane (GBM) [8, 10]. In the Burkholder variant, there were discrete subendothelial and subepithelial deposits (**Figure 2**), while in the Anders-Strife variant, the deposits produced complex transmembranous, ribbon-like subendothelial and subepithelial deposits with fraying of the lamina densa (**Figure 3**).

MPGN type II was first described by Berger and Galle in 1963 as a dense deposit disease (DDD) characterized by extremely electron dense transformation of the GBM (**Figure 4**) [11]. Little attention was paid to this entity until 1975, when Habib indicated an association between dense transformation of the GBM and the MPGN histologic pattern and therefore classified it as a type II variant of MPGN, which was followed by long-term consequences [12].

From the beginning, an MPGN lesion delineated a group of patients with no evidence of underlying disease—an idiopathic MPGN [9, 13]. Over time, as serological and other methodology improved, many secondary forms with clear etiologic associations were differentiated from idiopathic MPGN. It became apparent that MPGN is often associated with chronic infections (hepatitis B and C, with or without cryoglobulinemia), autoimmunity or deposition

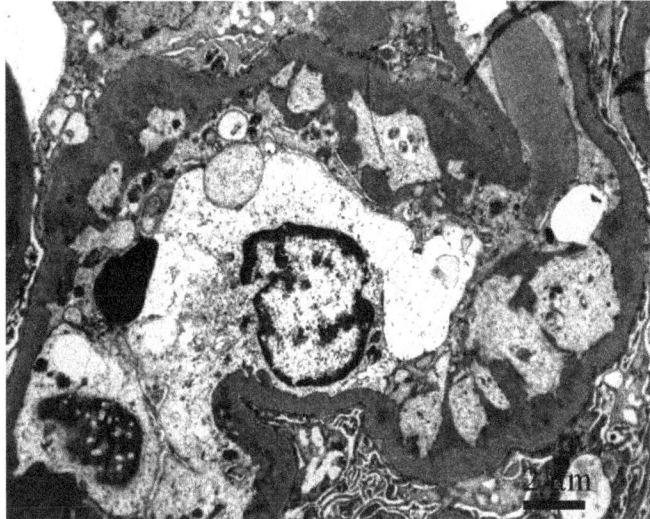

Figure 1. MPGN type I is characterized by mesangial and subendothelial deposits, with marked mesangial interposition and double contour formation.

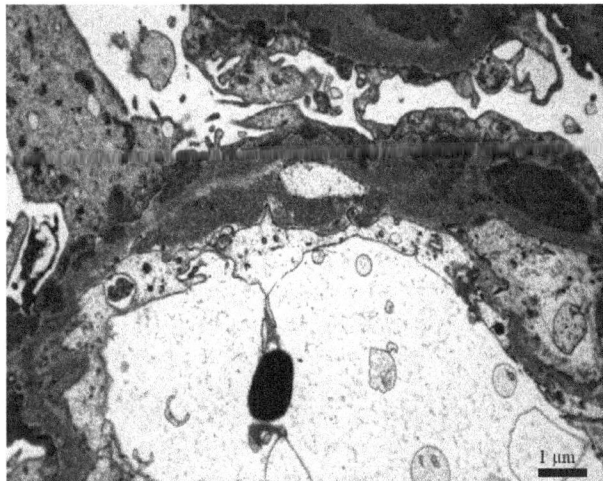

Figure 2. Burkholder variant of MPGN type III shows mesangial and discrete subendothelial and subepithelial deposits.

of a monoclonal immunoglobulin. A histologic pattern resembling the MPGN pattern could also be observed in a broad group of thrombotic microangiopathy: thrombotic thrombocytopenic purpura, atypical hemolytic uremic syndrome (aHUS), sickle cell anemia, diabetic glomerulosclerosis, transplant glomerulopathy and malignant hypertension [7, 14, 15]. In this group of diseases, there is little or no proliferation and neither marked mesangial interposition nor immune deposits are detected on immunofluorescence (IF) or EM. GBM double contours occur due to subendothelial neolamina formation in response to insudative changes, endothelial swelling and subendothelial plasma insudation.

This historical classification, based on histologic and ultrastructural findings and devoid of pathogenetic context, could not explain the diversity of underlying pathogenetic mechanisms, nor the various clinical pictures in MPGN patients [13]. It was tempting to speculate that other features, in addition to the peculiar description of deposits location, would clarify at least some group of

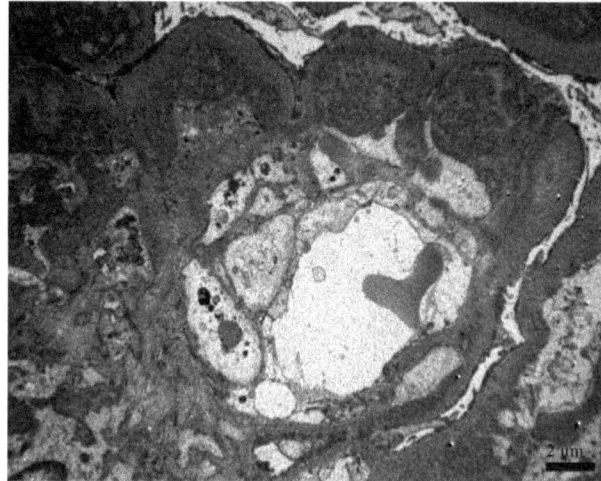

Figure 3. In Anders-Strife variant of MPGN type III, the deposits produce complex transmembranous, ribbon-like subendothelial, and subepithelial formations with fraying of the lamina densa.

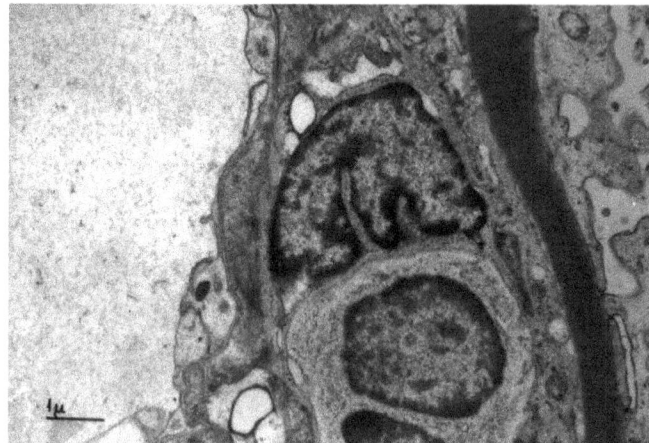

Figure 4. Highly electron dense intramembranous and mesangial deposits are hallmark of DDD, classified historically as MPGN type II.

patients with features of MPGN [14, 16, 17]. The discovery that many children with DDD displayed persistent hypocomplementemia, with low levels of serum complement factors, was a harbinger of the identification of the heterogeneity of mechanisms underlying the MPGN pattern [17].

It was increasingly observed that many patients with dense deposits on EM, characteristic of MPGN type II lacked a MPGN pattern on light microscopy [18]. In order to disprove the relation between dense transformation of GBM and a MPGN histologic pattern, Walker collected 69 cases of DDD from centers in North America, Europe and Japan [19].

Surprisingly, four histologic patterns were identified: membranoproliferative, mesangial proliferative, crescentic, and acute proliferative and exudative. The MPGN pattern was found only in 25% of cases; the majority of patients presented with mesangial proliferative features. On light microscopy and IF, the acute proliferative and exudative variants can be difficult to distinguish from post-infectious glomerulonephritis [20, 21].

Concurrently, improving IF techniques enabled differentiation of the composition of the deposits detected by IF [9, 22]. Biopsies from patients with MPGN type II usually showed only C3 deposits, with little or without immunoglobulin deposition. Furthermore, even in some cases of MPGN types I and III, pathologists noticed the presence of dominant complement deposits, therefore setting these cases apart from more common variants of type I and III containing immunoglobulins and C3. These cases were initially called idiopathic MPGN with dominant C3 deposits [13, 23]. Moreover, patients with MPGN and dominant C3 deposits also presented with low serum C3, indicating complement alternative pathway dysregulation, while serum levels of classical complement factors were mainly normal. Laser micro dissection and mass spectrometry data of glomeruli from DDD and MPGN with dominant C3 deposits showed a similar proteomic profile, indicating a common pathogenesis of the two diseases [24, 25]. A major breakthrough was the discovery of genetic mutations or deficiencies in complement regulatory proteins in patients with predominant C3 deposits [14, 26].

2.1. Proposal for a new classification

The aforementioned elucidations of the possible pathogenesis of MPGN led to a new classification based on the composition of deposits: into immune complex-mediated and complement-mediated diseases [2, 4, 5, 27, 28].

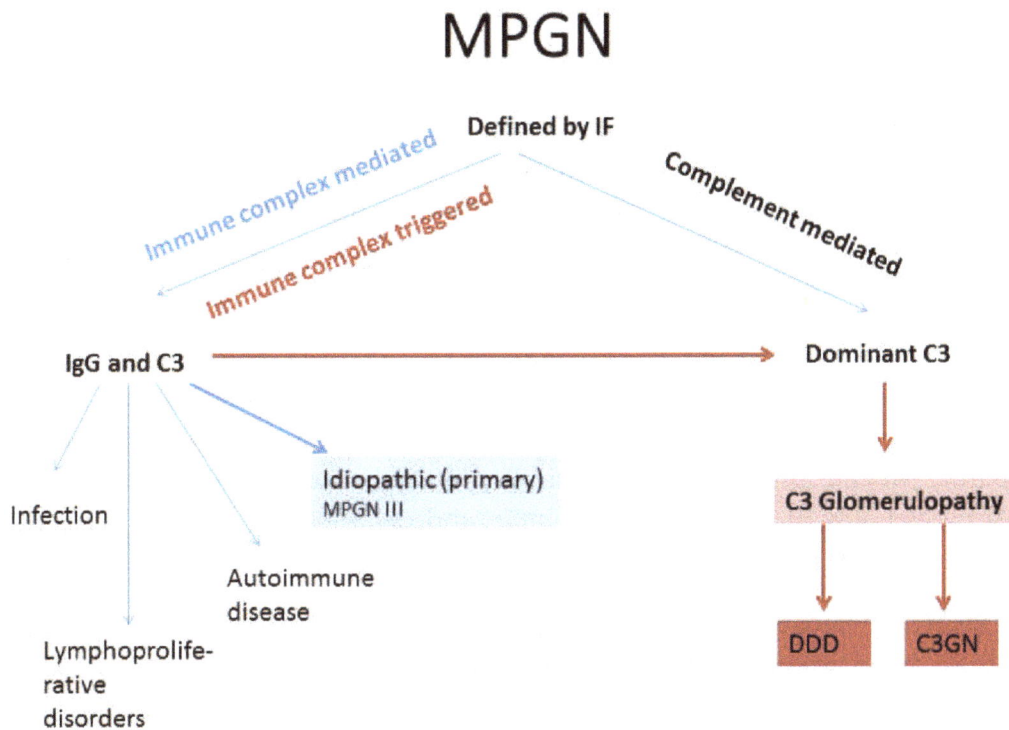

Figure 5. The evolving classification of MPGN: the composition of the deposits seen on IF categorized MPGN as immune complex-mediated and complement-mediated disease, the later termed C3 glomerulopathy. Immune complex-mediated MPGN without known underlying cause (idiopathic MPGN) may be immune complex-mediated at the beginning, evolving into C3 glomerulopathy over time. MPGN membranoproliferative glomerulonephritis, IF immunofluorescence.

Immune complex-mediated MPGN results from the deposition of immunoglobulin deposits and C3 driven by classical complement pathway activation, while complement-mediated disease may be associated with complement alternative pathway dysregulation and is a new entity, C3 glomerulopathy. C3 glomerulopathy is characterized by predominant C3 deposits on IF (**Figure 5**) [5, 9, 29].

C3 glomerulopathy is an umbrella term, encompassing DDD (former MPGN type II) and examples of MPGN types I and III, in which IF reveals exclusive or predominant C3 deposits, now termed C3 glomerulonephritis (C3GN) [4, 5, 22, 29, 30]. DDD is defined by the presence of dense osmiophilic transformation of the GBM on EM. Only EM enables definite distinction of DDD from C3GN; however, a spectrum of appearances may be seen in some cases, even in the same glomerulus.

3. Diagnosing C3 glomerulopathy

Cases with a membranoproliferative pattern that have only glomerular C3, with absolutely no immunoglobulin, are relatively uncommon; most cases will have dominant C3 staining with some immunoglobulin. The original definition of C3 glomerulopathy as "C3 only" appeared too stringent if the goal of diagnosis is to identify all complement-mediated cases for evaluation of complement alternative pathway dysregulation [2, 28, 30, 31].

In a study of over 300 cases of idiopathic MPGN, Hou et al. applied a hierarchical set of criteria to define the optimal cut-off for a diagnosis of C3 glomerulopathy, using DDD as a gold standard [22]. A new definition of C3 glomerulopathy was therefore proposed, for when C3 dominance is at least two orders of magnitude stronger than any other immune reactant. The new definition identified 31% of MPGN type 1, 88% of DDD (MPGN type II) and 39% of MPGN type III cases, indicating a sensitivity of 88% and acceptable specificity.

In terms of the modern approach to MPGN, 39% of the Anders-Strife variant would be classified as C3GN, whereas the majority of the Burkholder variant and approximately 70% of MPGN type I presented with immunoglobulin and C3 deposits as immune complex-mediated MPGN [22]. In many of those cases, an underlying cause could be identified, such as autoimmunity, chronic infection or deposition of a monoclonal immunoglobulin, indicating that idiopathic MPGN might now be considered a rare condition. It encompasses historical MPGN types I and III with immunoglobulin and complement deposits without known underlying cause [9, 31].

However, such rare cases might represent C3GN with immunoglobulin deposits, which did not fulfill the diagnostic criteria for C3 glomerulopathy at the time of diagnosis, and therefore an underlying complement dysregulation has to be excluded [31, 32].

It has already been proposed that, in some patients, immune complexes may initiate MPGN, but the disease is accelerated and sustained by complement alternative pathway dysregulation [30]. When a complement activating infection occurs, it may overwhelm the compensatory regulatory mechanisms, leading to augmented and perpetuated activation of dysregulated complement alternative pathway. MPGN may therefore be immune complex-mediated at the beginning, evolving into C3 glomerulopathy over time (**Figure 5**).

Although the proposed classification seems to be widely accepted, a recent study indicates that understanding MPGN by classification into immunoglobulin-mediated and C3 dominant forms might be too simplistic and may not provide sufficient information on prognosis and prevention of the disease [33]. In the future, novel research methods, probably based on mathematical models, will be employed in order to provide detailed insights into management of C3 glomerulopathy [33].

4. Dense deposit disease

4.1. Clinical presentation

DDD is a rare disease, with a reported incidence between 2 and 3 per million of the population, primarily affecting children and young adults, although the range is broad, varying from 1 to 64 years [19]. Recently, a study with the largest American cohort to date, including 111 patients with C3 glomerulopathy, 24 of them with DDD, found 29% of patients older than 50 years [3]. Males and females are usually equally involved, but some studies have reported a female predominance [1].

The clinical presentation is usually unspecific, with a slow deterioration of renal function. In the past, approximately 50% of patients presented with nephrotic syndrome at the time of diagnosis [12, 34, 35]. A recent study showed that most patients displayed proteinuria and hematuria with preserved kidney function, although about 25% of patients showed significant chronic kidney disease at the time of diagnosis [3]. Acute, often a respiratory tract infection prior to DDD onset was reported in approximately half of the patients, and this did not differ between pediatric and adult populations [1, 3, 12]. Progression to ESRD has been reported in up to 50% of patients within 10 years of diagnosis [2, 36].

Approximately 65–80% of patients with DDD present with persistently low serum C3 but serum levels of the early classic pathway components C1q and C4 are usually normal [1–3, 12]. Pediatric patients had lower C3 levels than adults [1, 3]. Up to 80% of patients with DDD showed positive serum C3 nephritic factor (C3Nef), an autoantibody directed against alternative pathway convertase, although it is not specific and is also found in patients with MPGN type I, post-infectious glomerulonephritis and even lupus nephritis [2, 35, 37–40]. Other autoantibodies against complement factors, including anti factor H antibody, anti-factor B antibody and complement factor gene variant and mutations have been found in various percentages of DDD patients [2, 3].

Rarely, patients with DDD may present with two other conditions, either separately or together: ocular drusen or acquired partial lipodystrophy. Both conditions are associated with dysregulation of the alternative complement pathway [14, 19, 41].

Ocular drusen are yellow deposits localized between the retinal pigment epithelium and Bruch's membrane, consisting of lipoproteinaceous deposits of complement-containing debris [42, 43]. Similar drusen are found in patients with age-related macular degeneration (AMD) but in contrast to patients with AMD, drusen in DDD patients occur at an early age. The same polymorphisms in factor H have been identified in patients with AMD and DDD, implicating AP complement dysregulation in the pathogenesis of both diseases [41, 44].

DDD can be rarely associated with acquired partial lipodystrophy (APL), the symmetrical loss of subcutaneous fat in the upper half of the body (face, arms and upper part of the trunk) [45]. Approximately 20% of patients with APL develop MPGN. APL usually precedes the onset of kidney disease by several years. Frequent detection of C3Nef and low C3 level in these patients indicates an underlying dysregulation of AP complement on both kidneys and adipose tissue. The deposition of activated complement factors in adipose tissue may result in the destruction of adipocytes [45].

4.2. Pathologic findings

4.2.1. Light microscopy

A specific feature of DDD is the presence of dense osmiophilic transformation of the GBM on EM [19, 20]. Due to the association between dense GBM transformation and an MPGN histological pattern described decades ago, it was classified historically as MPGN type II [12]. However, the appearance of DDD on light microscopy is quite variable, showing membrano-proliferative, mesangial proliferative, crescentic and acute proliferative, and exudative histologic patterns [1, 20]. In some cases, glomeruli show prominent endocapillary hypercellularity with exudation of neutrophils reminiscent of post-infectious glomerulonephritis, while others present with a prominent crescent formation. In an American cohort of 24 patients, membranoproliferative and mesangial patterns were demonstrated in 46 and 29% of patients, respectively [3]. The clinical significance of the different patterns needs further evaluation, but in some patients, it might depend on the timing of the biopsy; patients with long-lasting disease may develop chronic glomerular changes with double contours characteristic of a membranoproliferative pattern.

On light microscopy, GBM dense deposits are recognized as thickening of the glomerular capillary walls by ribbon-like intramembranous deposits. They are intensely periodic acid-Schiff (PAS) positive and stain strongly fuchsinophilic (red) with trichrome stain. Methenamine silver staining discloses characteristic defects in the GBM because dense deposits are not argyrophilic and therefore fail to stain with silver stains. Thin, silver-positive lines border the GBM on each side, resulting in typical double contours (**Figure 6**). Although light microscopy in typical cases is fairly characteristic, the glomerular intramembranous deposits may vary in size and number and a definitive diagnosis can be established only by EM [20, 32].

4.2.2. Immunofluorescence

DDD is characterized by the presence of intense C3 deposits in the glomerular mesangium, as well as along capillary walls, with minimal or no immunoglobulin deposition. There are usually abundant mesangial C3 deposits, described as coarse granules, spherules or small rings (**Figure 7**). The IF pattern along the glomerular capillary walls is described as pseudolinear,

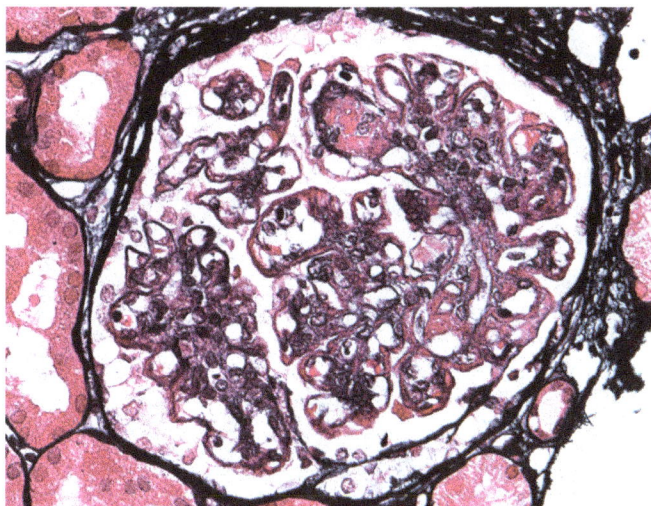

Figure 6. Extensive mesangial deposits and thickening of the glomerular capillary walls by ribbon-like intramembranous deposits. Deposits stain strongly fuchsinophilic (red) with trichrome stain. Methenamine silver staining discloses characteristic defects in the GBM. (silver and trichrome stain—Jones and Azan, 400×).

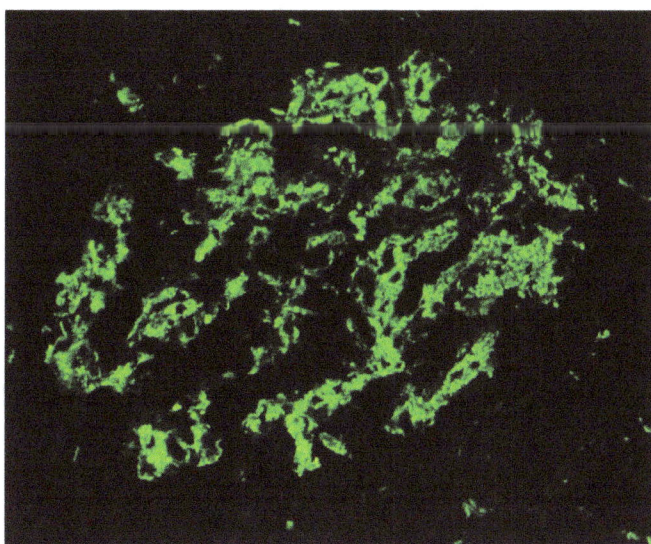

Figure 7. Intense ring-like C3 deposits in the glomerular mesangium and pseudolinear along capillary walls in DDD.

smooth, ribbon-like or coarsely granular. Classical complement components and immunoglobulin staining are usually absent; if present, they stain less intensely than C3 and may be focal and segmental [20, 34]. C3 deposits may be also found in the basal lamina of the Bowman capsule and along the tubular basement membranes of proximal and distal tubules.

4.2.3. Electron microscopy

DDD is characterized by the presence of dense transformation of the GBM found by EM. This special appearance of the lamina densa may be continuous and diffuse in distribution (**Figure 4**) or interrupted and fusiform, with native GBM found between deposits (**Figure 8**). In less severe cases, dense deposits may be focal, affecting only a few loops. The deposits

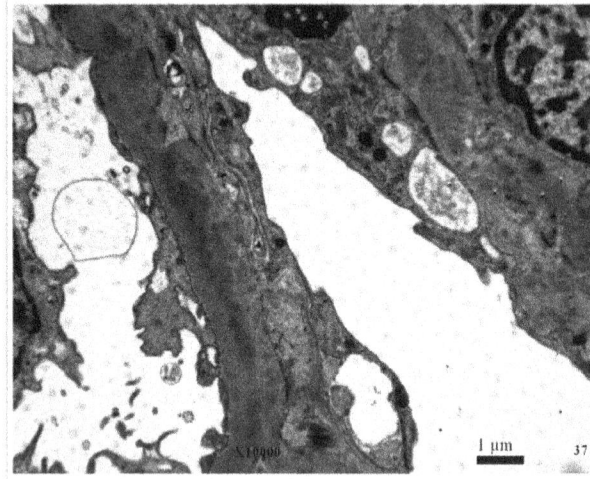

Figure 8. In less extensive cases of DDD deposits occupy only part of the GBM width.

may replace the entire width of the lamina densa, whereas in less extensive involvement they occupy only part of the GBM width (**Figure 8**). Mild cases may present only in the inner (subendothelial) aspect of the GBM. Subendothelial electron dense deposits sometimes evolve to more hyaline transmembrane deposits, with a lower electron density found in C3GN [18, 20, 34]. Many patients show subepithelial electron dense deposits, in some cases reminiscent of hump-like deposits seen in post-infectious glomerulonephritis.

In addition to glomerular deposits, electron dense transformation has been described in the basement membrane of Bowman's capsule and renal tubules, although usually focal and segmental [1, 12, 19, 34]. Dense electron change has also been found in the afferent arterioles and the area of the macula densa [12].

It is noteworthy that drusen, a characteristic pathologic finding in the Bruch's membrane in patients with DDD, and macular degeneration have the same ultrastructural appearance as the GBM in DDD [42]. Except for a report of electron dense transformation in the sinusoidal BM of the spleen in two patients with DDD, in no other organ systems have similar electron dense deposits been identified so far [46, 47].

The exact ultrastructure of electron dense deposits and the mechanism of unique GBM transformation remain to be elucidated. The three-dimensional ultrastructural findings of GBM in DDD patients suggest rigid and thickened GBM with a coarsely granular or undulating surface punctuated by single or clustered crater-like deformities unique to DDD [48].

5. C3 glomerulonephritis

C3 glomerulonephritis is characterized by exclusive or predominant C3 deposits on IF and electron dense mesangial and glomerular capillary walls deposits on EM, without electron dense osmiophilic transformation of the GBM characteristic of DDD. It encompasses examples of historical MPGN types I and III and other histological patterns in which IF reveals dominant C3 deposits, indicating complement alternative pathway dysregulation as the underlying pathogenetic mechanism [24].

5.1. Clinical presentation

C3GN is a heterogeneous disease with respect to pathogenesis, clinical course and prognosis. Numerous mutations and polymorphisms in genes that code for proteins involved in complement alternative pathway and acquired abnormalities have been identified in patients with C3GN. There are two examples of familial forms of the disease with specific mutations, including CFHR5 nephropathy endemic in Cyprus and familial MPGN from Ireland [49, 50].

A recent study of a diverse American cohort including 111 patients with C3 glomerulopathy provided detailed information on the clinical presentation of C3GN and DDD [3]. Whites comprised the majority of C3GN patients (63.2%), followed by Hispanic, Asian and African-American patients, accounting for 19.5, 12.6 and 4.6% of the cohort, respectively. Surprisingly, patients with C3GN (mean age 28.3) were significantly younger than patients with DDD (mean age 40.0 years). The most common clinical presentation was hematuria and proteinuria with normal kidney function in both groups, but chronic kidney disease with proteinuria and hematuria was more frequent in DDD patients (41.7% in DDD vs. 18.6% in C3GN). Patients with C3GN more often presented with nephrotic syndrome than did DDD patients (32.6 vs. 16.7%). The prevalence of low complement level was the same in both groups, although the pediatric population demonstrated a significantly higher prevalence of low C3 levels and twice the rate of detectable genetic variants and/or autoantibodies.

Progression to end-stage renal disease (ESRD) was found in 40% of C3G patients, with no detectable difference between those with C3GN versus DDD, although previous reports have suggested a more favorable clinical course in C3GN patients [2, 26, 51, 52]. Markers of chronicity, whether clinical (reduced estimated glomerular filtration rate (eGFR), elevated serum creatinine) or histologic (interstitial fibrosis, glomerulosclerosis) at the time of diagnosis appeared the strongest predictors of outcome.

5.2. Pathologic findings

5.2.1. Light microscopy

C3GN is defined by dominant C3 deposits on IF and deposits on EM. The light microscopic features are variable, including mesangial proliferation, a membranoproliferative pattern, crescent formation and endocapillary hypercellularity (**Figures 9–11**). There is no known association of the various histologic patterns with the underlying genetic or functional abnormalities of complement dysregulation [3, 24].

Bomback proposed a C3 Glomerulopathy Histologic Index to score biopsy activity and chronicity, in order to determine predictors of progression to ESRD in patients with C3GN [3, 24]. The activity score included mesangial hypercellularity, endocapillary hypercellularity, membranoproliferative morphology, leukocyte infiltration, crescent formation, fibrinoid necrosis and interstitial inflammation, while the chronicity score encompassed

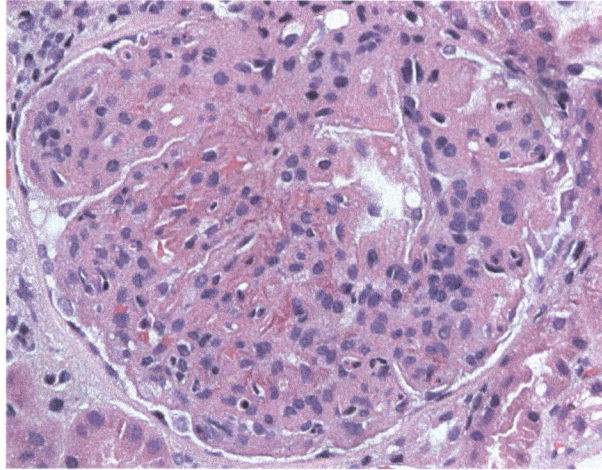

Figure 9. C3GN with membranoproliferative pattern (HE, 400×).

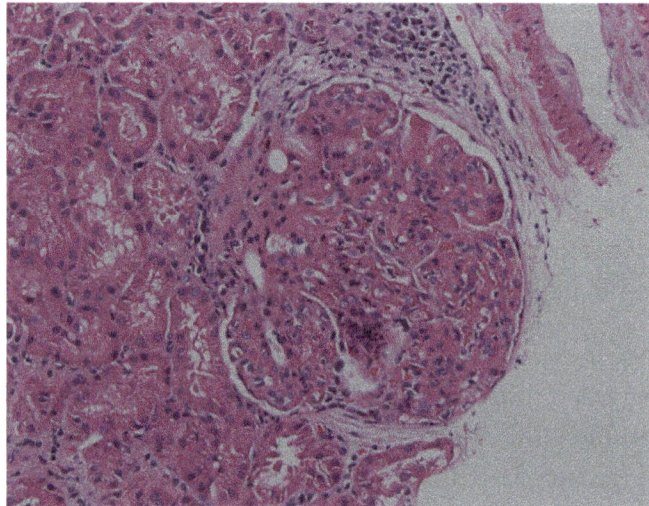

Figure 10. C3GN with membranoproliferative pattern with exudation of neutrophils (HE, 200×).

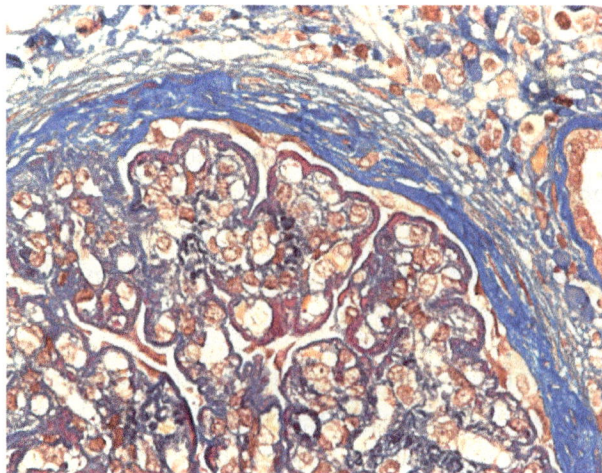

Figure 11. C3GN with membranoproliferative pattern with abundant transmembranous deposits staining with trichrome stain reminiscent of DDD (Trichrome stain, 600×).

glomerulosclerosis, tubular atrophy/interstitial fibrosis and arterio-arteriolosclerosis. Patients with C3GN showed a higher activity score than DDD patients, and the latter revealed a higher chronicity score. In multivariable models, the strongest predictors of progression were eGFR at the time of diagnosis and tubular atrophy/interstitial fibrosis. The C3 Glomerulopathy Histologic Index might emerge as a useful tool for predicting the prognosis and management of patients with C3 glomerulopathy [3].

5.2.2. Immunofluorescence

The defining feature on IF is the presence of dominant C3 glomerular deposits, at least two orders of magnitude stronger than any other immune reactant. It is noteworthy that a proposed cut-off does not encompass all patients with alternative pathway dysregulation, and there are overlaps between C3GN and immune complex glomerulonephritis [27, 29, 31].

In cases presenting with a mesangial histological pattern, C3 staining is mainly mesangial, while in the membranoproliferative pattern, there are abundant capillary wall as well as mesangial C3 deposits. In some cases, C3 staining was also found on the TBM [24, 53].

5.2.3. Electron microscopy

EM revealed electron dense deposits in the mesangium and along or within the GBM, which correspond to C3 deposits on IF. Consistent with the definition of C3 glomerulopathy, deposits are composed predominantly of complement factors, although they may show similar density and appear at the same locations as deposits composed of immunoglobulins and C3 [24]. In some cases, deposits may be less dense and less sharply demarcated than typical immune complex deposits (**Figure 12**). In the glomerular capillary walls, there are abundant transmembrane deposits that appear to replace areas of the lamina densa, separated by material of similar density as the lamina densa, similar to the Anders Strife variant of MPGN type III (**Figure 13**). In some cases, there are curvilinear deposits of more electron dense material in the mesangium and

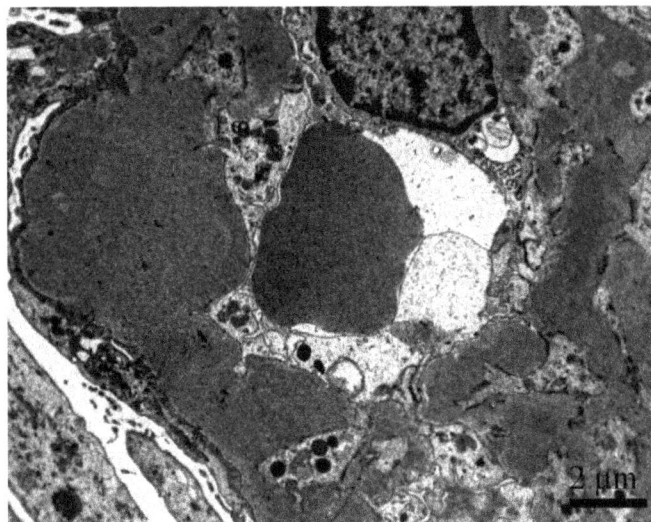

Figure 12. Abundant transmembrane deposits in C3GN may be less dense and less sharply demarcated than typical immune complex deposits.

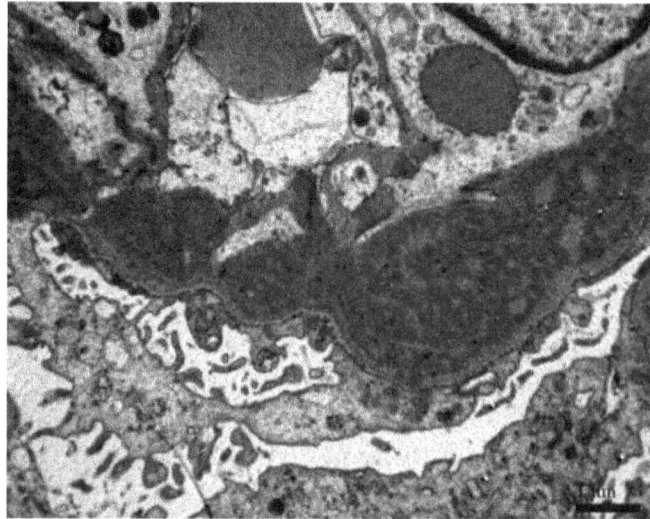

Figure 13. Abundant transmembrane deposits that replace areas of the lamina densa, separated by material of similar density as the lamina densa, similar to the Anders Strife variant of MPGN type III.

beneath the endothelium, reminiscent of deposits in DDD. Occasional cases display substantial overlapping features between DDD and C3GN, making the subcategorization difficult [32].

Many C3GN patients present with subepithelial deposits. They may sometimes appear as subepithelial projections of intramembranous deposits but, in some cases, they resemble typical subepithelial humps seen in post-infectious glomerulonephritis. It is tempting to speculate that they may be related to C3GN exacerbated by infections [21].

6. Overview of the complement system

The complement system is a complex cascade in which proteolytic cleavage of glycoproteins induces an inflammatory response, phagocyte chemotaxis, opsonization, and cell lysis. It is triggered through three different pathways: the classical, alternative and mannose binding lectin, which converge on C3 to form an enzyme complex C3 convertase. C3 convertase cleaves C3, generating C3a, an anaphylatoxin, and C3b, a potent opsonin. A positive feedback loop, termed the C3 amplification loop, enables rapid amplification of C3b, which can generate millions of C3b molecules. C3b then deposit on cell surfaces, triggering complement cascade activation. Through the binding of an additional C3b molecule, C3 convertase becomes C5 convertase (C3bBbBB), which is capable of cleaving complement C5 into C5a and C5b. C5b, through sequential interaction with complements C6, C7, C8 and C9, generates membrane attack complex (MAC) [32, 54, 55].

In contrast to classical and lectin pathways, the alternative pathway is continually active in the circulation, by spontaneous hydrolysis of an internal thioester bond in C3 (thick over mechanism). Hydrolyzed C3 interacts with complement factor B (CFB) to form C3iB. CFB within C3iB is cleaved by complement factor D, resulting in C3 convertase (C3iBb), which cleaves C3 to a small amount of C3b. Cleaved C3b, similar to C3i, interacts with complement factors B to form C3 convertase (C3bBbBB). If the generation of C3 is not tightly regulated, it can be rapidly amplified through a positive feedback pathway (C3b amplification loop), which results in activation of downstream convertase C5 and MAC formation. Several complement degradation products, including iC3b, are delivered to the endothelial surfaces, including the glomeruli. The deposition of complement products in the mesangium and in the subendothelial region triggers glomerular inflammation, leading to GN, often with a MPGN pattern [32].

Complement regulation is achieved by complement activator proteins and regulatory proteins present in plasma (fluid phase) and on cell surfaces (solid phase). Both regulate complement activation at different steps and pathways. If complement activator proteins are deficient, there is too little complement and these patients predispose to infections and autoimmune diseases. In regulatory protein deficiency, the complement system is upregulated, which results in impaired regulation and too much complement. Due to spontaneous activation of the alternative pathway and potency of the C3b amplification loop, both pathways are tightly regulated by complement factor I (CFI) and complement factor H (CFH) [30, 56].

Fluid phase regulators include factors CFH and CFI, whereas decay accelerating factor (DAF, CD55), complement receptor 1, CD 59 and membrane cofactor protein (MCP), are cell-bound regulators that act on cell surfaces [30]. Dysregulation between activating and regulatory factors in the fluid phase results in permanent activation of C3 convertase and at least partial activation of downstream complement factors, including C5 convertase and other proteins of the terminal complement cascade.

6.1. Complement factor I

CFI is a serine protease that cleaves C3b to iC3b and C3. While C3b can form C3 convertase, iC3b and C3d cannot, so the CFI-mediated cleavage of C3b stops further C3b activation. CFI can cleave C3b in the presence of cofactors, including CFH, membrane-bound protein (CD 46) and complement receptor 1 (CR1, CD35). In CFI deficiency, the spontaneous activation of the AP and, consequently, C3b amplification continue uncontrolled, leading to severe depletion of C3 in the plasma. Because CFI is crucial for generation of iC3b, iC3b cannot arise in complete CFI deficiency. Mice models have shown that the presence of CFI is crucial for deposits in the GBM and these deposits might be in the form of iC3b [30].

6.2. Complement factor H

Plasma protein CFH is the major negative regulator of the complement alternative pathway synthetized predominantly in the liver. It regulates C3 activation in two different compartments: in plasma (fluid phase) and along surfaces (solid phase) [32].

CFH is composed of 20 short consensus repeat (SCR) domains, with two major binding sites. The first four amino terminal domains represent binding sites for C3 convertase, thus regulating C3 in the fluid phase. The last two carboxyl terminal domains are involved in C3 activation along surfaces (solid phase) [30].

In plasma, CFH regulates C3 activation in different ways: it blocks the formation of AP convertase by binding to C3b, in order to inhibit interaction between C3b and factor B. Second, it accelerates the spontaneous breakdown of AP C3 convertase and is a cofactor for CFI mediated inactivation of C3b to iC3b [32]. CFH deficiency results in uncontrolled C3b generation and secondary C3 depletion, but generation of C3b, iC3b and C3d is possible. In contrast, in complete CFI deficiency, generation of iC3b and C3d cannot occur.

CFH also regulates C3 activation along surfaces, including the renal endothelium and GBM. Optimal functioning of CFH requires interaction with C3b and polyanions. Through the terminal two carboxyl terminal domains, CFH attaches to cell surfaces and extracellular membranes, adding a protective mechanism to prevent complement activity on cell surfaces.

CFH is therefore involved in both fluid phase and solid phase regulation and mutation on different binding sites of the same regulatory protein may lead to different diseases. Mutations that selectively affect C3 regulation domains are associated with C3 glomerulopathy, whereas those affecting surface recognition domains are responsible for aHUS. In aHUS, there is complement-mediated damage to the renal endothelium, with consequent development of thrombotic microangiopathy [30, 56, 57].

Mice models provide some insights into the pathogenesis of aHUS and DDD. CFH mutations in aHUS affect predominantly the carboxyl terminal domains, resulting in impaired surface regulation, but the ability to regulate plasma C3 convertase is preserved. If the mutation affects the amino terminal domains, uncontrolled fluid phase C3 convertase activation occurs, resulting in disease analogous to DDD. Therefore, in DDD, the critical step is activation of C3 convertase in the fluid phase. In aHUS, the critical step is activation of C5 convertase and impaired surface regulation at the level of the cell membrane, in the solid phase. This solid phase dysregulation makes aHUS a more homogeneous disease than C3 glomerulopathy, with implications for prognosis and response to therapy [57].

6.3. Complement factor H-related proteins 1–5

There are five genes adjacent to the CFH gene, which encode structurally related proteins complement factor H-related proteins 1–5 (CFHR1–5). There are many regions of sequence homology across the CFH-CFHR locus that, through recombination, enables structural variations of CFHR: partial deletion or whole gene deletion or duplication, implying that these proteins are biologically redundant. Several combined deletions of different CFHR are found in various frequencies in a healthy population. The most common variant is combined deletion of the CFHR1 and CFHR3 genes, presenting in 5 and 16% of Caucasian and African-American populations, respectively [50].

Polymorphic variations within the CFH-CFHR gene locus are associated with diverse pathologies, including age-related macular degeneration (AMD), meningococcal sepsis, thrombotic and inflammatory kidney diseases such as aHUS and C3 glomerulopathy, and autoimmune diseases. The significance of homozygous deletion of CFHR1, 3 genes and the mechanisms of action are poorly understood. It might increase the risk of developing SLE, but is protective to IgA nephropathy and AMD, pathologies associated with complement deposition in affected tissues [41, 58, 59]. Based on a protective role for CFHR1, 3 genes deletion in IgA nephropathy, Malik et al. developed the hypothesis that the presence of CFHR1, 3 proteins impairs complement processing within the kidney [50].

6.3.1. The role of CFHR5 in complement regulation

Previous reports based on in vitro studies have implicated the involvement of CFHR proteins in complement regulatory activity [60]. According to a recent approach, these proteins have no direct complement regulatory activity at physiologic concentrations, unlike CFH [32].

The investigators postulated that CFHR5 may compete with CFH for binding to activated C3b. If CFH binds, C3b is inactivated, preventing further complement activation. Conversely, if CFHR binds to activated C3b, this prevents CFH binding, therefore enabling C3 convertase formation and continued complement activation. Since these proteins are devoid of intrinsic regulatory complement activity, this has been termed CFH deregulation [61].

CFHR1, CFHR2, and CFHR5 have recently been shown to form homodimers and heterodimers via common dimerization domains within SCR1 and SCR2 [62]. The dimerization of CFHR1, CFHR2 and CFHR5 may enhance the avidity of these proteins for ligand in vivo, thereby preventing CFH binding and thus functioning as complement deregulators [62].

The deregulation hypothesis could also explain the protective effect of CFHR1, 3 genes deletion in IgA nephropathy. Fewer CFHRs in serum could lead to less CFH deregulation, enabling tighter control of complement activation and inflammation. Conversely, circulating CFHR proteins 1 and 5 may correlate with increased disease activity, as shown in a large cohort of patients with IgA nephropathy [63].

6.4. Membrane cofactor protein

MCP is a surface-bound complement regulatory protein acting as a cofactor for the CFI mediated cleavage of C3b to iC3b on the cell surface. Polymorphism in the promoter region may influence MCP expression at the cell surfaces, which may explain the various patterns of deposits in C3G [2]. The majority of mutations in CD46 are detected in the extracellular domains of CD46 responsible for C3b and C4b binding.

7. Familiar forms of C3 glomerulopathy

7.1. CFHR5 nephropathy

Heterozygous mutations in CFHR5 are characteristic findings in complement factor H-related protein 5 nephropathy (CFHR5 nephropathy) [49, 64]. CFHR5 nephropathy is a subtype of C3GN, with autosomal dominant inheritance discovered in Cypriot families. A heterozygous mutation in CFHR5 results in duplication of the first two protein subunits, termed short consensus repeat. Affected individuals possess both the wild-type nine-domain CFHR5 protein and an abnormally large mutant CFHR5, with 11 domains [64].

Clinically, patients present with microscopic hematuria, proteinuria and synpharyngitic macroscopic hematuria similar to IgA nephropathy. There is progression to end-stage renal disease over the age of 50, particularly in males. Renal biopsies show deposition of C3 in the mesangium, and characteristic elongated subendothelial electron dense deposits, and occasional subepithelial deposits. The laboratory profile of patients is normal, without decreased C3 levels, indicating that the complement activation occurs locally in the kidney and not at a systemic level. It has been speculated that abnormal CFHR5 in CFHR5 nephropathy may prevent CFH mediated regulation of C3, leading to increased activation of C3 along the glomerular basement membrane [64].

7.2. Other familiar forms of C3 glomerulonephritis

Recently, an abnormal CFHR5 protein in a family without Cypriot ancestry, identical to the aberrant CFHR5 protein found in Cypriot CFHR5 nephropathy, was identified, related to familial C3 glomerulonephritis. The clinical characteristics of the nephropathy in this pedigree were remarkably similar to Cypriot CFHR5 nephropathy: the typical presentation was with microscopic and intermittent macroscopic hematuria, and renal disease was more severe in affected males [65]. The genomic rearrangement was distinct from that seen in Cypriot CFHR5 nephropathy, although identical protein was identified.

A duplication of SCR 1–4 of CFHR1 was revealed in another familial form of C3G [66]. In mutant CFHR1, duplication of the N-terminal domain resulted in the formation of unusually large multimeric CFHR complexes that exhibited enhanced binding of mutated CFHR1 to ligands C3b, iC3b and C3d, resulting in enhanced competition and replacement of CFH bound to C3b. Patients usually presented with decreased C3 plasma levels, suggesting fluid phase complement activation and systemic disease.

8. Genetic and acquired abnormalities of complement associated with C3 glomerulopathy

C3G is associated with genetic and acquired abnormalities that result in uncontrolled activation of the complement alternative pathway. With the exception of diacilglicerol kinase epsilon, all genes associated with C3 glomerulopathy encode proteins in the complement system [67]. Mutations in complement factors and complement regulators are rare, but certain genetic polymorphisms contributing to fine balancing of complement regulation are more common.

Due to the complexity of the disease, C3 glomerulopathy is rarely inherited in a simple Mendelian fashion [68]. Rare familial cases of C3 glomerulopathy comprise highly penetrant heterozygous copy number variants involving CFHR1–5 genes described in Cypriot families, a family of Irish ancestry and a recently described family of non-Cypriot origin [49, 65, 66].

Most pathogenic variants of the C3 gene affect the proper cleavage of C3 protein by affecting recognition sites for binding of CFH or CFI. Loss-of-function changes in CFH, gain-of-function changes in C3 and structural changes within the CFH-CFHR gene family have been identified [69].

Acquired abnormalities include antibodies to complement activating proteins, such as antibody to C3 convertase, and antibodies which target the inhibitory complement factors

(CFH or CFI autoantibodies). C3Nef, antibody to C3 convertase, stabilizes C3 convertase of the alternative pathway by preventing its inactivation and degradation. Recent studies have shown that some autoantibodies might arise due to underlying genetic abnormalities [68].

In the largest study to date, encompassing 134 patients, Servais et al. analyzed the presence of C3Nef and other genetic and acquired abnormalities in patients with DDD, C3GN and primary MPGN type I [2]. C3Nef was identified in 86% of patients with DDD, but it was also present in 24% of GNC3 patients and even in 53% of patients with primary MPGN type I. CFH mutations were found in a similar frequency in all three groups of patients. MCP mutations seem to be very rare, identified in only one patient with C3GN. Another very interesting report described three patients with known homozygous CFH deficiency, who presented with different histological patterns, varying from mesangial proliferative to membranoproliferative [70]. Studies from rare cases with known genetic abnormalities indicate that entities with predominant C3 deposits, DDD and C3GN, as well as immune complex MPGN, are heterogeneous diseases.

Genetic or acquired complement AP abnormalities have also been identified in association with immune complex-mediated glomerulonephritis, such as systemic lupus erythematosus, and particularly frequently in patients with immune complex-mediated MPGN and atypical post-infectious glomerulonephritis, the latter showing overlapping features with C3 glomerulopathy [2, 21]. The question of why some patients present with DDD while others with ill-defined intramembranous deposits consistent with C3GN remains to be answered. The processes driving the particular morphologic appearance of glomerular deposits seem to be very complex, including genetic and environmental factors.

9. Treatment in C3 glomerulopathy

There is no universally effective treatment for C3 glomerulopathy. The only double blind randomized control trial was performed on 80 children with MPGN types I, II and III in 1992. They received 40 mg/m^2 of prednisolone on alternate days. Long-term treatment with prednisolone appeared to improve the outcome of patients with MPGN [71]. Other studies have suggested some benefit from the use of cyclophosphamide, mycophenolate mofetil and a combination of aspirin and dipyridamole. Current guidelines suggest treatment with steroids and cytotoxic agents, with or without plasmapheresis, only in patients with progressive disease with nephrotic range proteinuria and a decline of renal function [72]. Because C3G is a new diagnostic category, long-term data on renal transplants are lacking, but recurrence is probably as high as in idiopathic MPGN type I (up to 65% in some series).

Rituximab has emerged in the last decade as a treatment option for patients with various primary glomerular diseases. Despite data on the use of rituximab in MPGN and C3G being limited, patients with immunoglobulin-associated and idiopathic MPGN treated with rituximab showed a partial or complete response in the majority of cases [72]. It can be hypothesized that, in the presence of autoantibodies such as C3Nef, B-cell depleting therapy may have led to decreased production of C3Nef and, subsequently, stable renal function [72]. However, rituximab was not effective in a few reported cases of C3GN and DDD. Only one patient with DDD and positive C3Nef treated solely with rituximab showed stable renal function and improvement of nephrotic syndrome after 30 months of follow-up, but C3Nef remained positive and C3 levels were always low [73]. In contrast, other cases with DDD and C3G initially treated with rituximab achieved partial or complete remission on eculizumab [72, 74].

Eculizumab is a humanized monoclonal antibody that binds with high affinity to C5 and prevents the generation of MAC and release of the very potent inflammatory mediator C5a. It is the treatment of choice in aHUS and paroxysmal nocturnal hematuria, but it may also provide an effective targeted treatment for patients with C3GN sharing an abnormality in the regulation of complement AP [75]. However, it has been suggested that eculizumab might be effective in some cases of C3GN, and that elevation of sMAC, lower circulating C3, short disease duration, acute lesions and limited fibrosis before treatment may predict a favorable response [24, 31, 76]. Eculizumab seems also to be effective in the treatment of a recurrence of DDD on renal transplants [76].

In patients with immune complex-mediated MPGN, refractory to conventional immunosuppression, the presence of complement AP dysregulation should be considered. When special laboratory and molecular genetic tests reveal an underlying complement alternative pathway dysregulation, they might respond to eculizumab treatment. Due to an initial immune complex-mediated mechanism, which can mask an underlying complement alternative pathway abnormality and subsequently trigger unbalanced excessive complement terminal pathway activation, supplementary steroids, in addition to eculizumab, may be necessary to achieve an adequate response [53].

10. Conclusions

C3 glomerulopathy is a heterogeneous disease, recently defined by dominant C3 glomerular deposits on immunofluorescence suggesting dysregulation of the alternative complement pathway as the underlying pathogenetic mechanism. It encompasses C3GN and DDD; DDD is characterized by dense osmiophilic deposits on EM. The appearance on light microscopy is quite variable, showing membranoproliferative, mesangial proliferative, crescentic, and acute proliferative and exudative histologic patterns. Genetic or acquired complement AP abnormalities have been identified in up to 40% of patients with C3 glomerulopathy, including mutations in complement factors or autoantibodies directed against them. Various clinical courses and histological features among patients with the same genetic defect indicate that other genetic factors or triggers from the environment contribute to the initiation and progression of complement mediated diseases. Despite multiple genetic risk factors, glomerular injury due to complement dysregulation often develops late in life, suggesting that additional triggers are required.

Acknowledgements

I would like to thank Jerica Pleško for performing electron microscopy examinations and electron micrographs.

Conflict of interest

There is nothing to declare.

Author details

Nika Kojc

Address all correspondence to: nika.kojc@mf.uni-lj.si

Institute of Pathology, Faculty of Medicine, University of Ljubljana, Ljubljana, Slovenia

References

[1] Nasr SH, Valeri AM, Appel GB, Sherwinter J, Stokes MB, Said SM, et al. Dense deposit disease: Clinicopathologic study of 32 pediatric and adult patients. Clinical Journal of the American Society of Nephrology. 2009;**4**:22-32

[2] Servais A, Noël LH, Roumenina LT, Le Quintrec M, Ngo S, Dragon-Durey MA, et al. Acquired and genetic complement abnormalities play a critical role in dense deposit disease and other C3 glomerulopathies. Kidney International. 2012;**82**:454-464

[3] Bomback AS, Santoriello D, Avasare RS, Regunathan-Shenk R, Canetta PA, Ahn W, et al. C3 glomerulonephritis and dense deposit disease share a similar disease course in a large United States cohort of patients with C3 glomerulopathy. Kidney International. 2018;**93**:977-985

[4] Sethi S, Fervenza FC. Membranoproliferative glomerulonephritis: Pathogenetic heterogeneity and proposal for a new classification. Seminars in Nephrology. 2011;**31**:341-348

[5] Sethi S, Fervenza FC. Membranoproliferative glomerulonephritis—A new look at an old entity. The New England Journal of Medicine. 2012;**366**:1119-1131

[6] Sethi S, Fervenza FC, Zhang Y, Nasr SH, Leung N, Vrana J, et al. Proliferative glomerulonephritis secondary to dysfunction of the alternative pathway of complement. Clinical Journal of the American Society of Nephrology. 2011;**6**:1009-1017

[7] Rennke HG. Secondary membranoproliferative glomerulonephritis. Kidney International. 1995;**47**:643-656

[8] Strife CF, McEnery PT, McAdams AJ, West CD. Membranoproliferative glomerulonephritis with disruption of the glomerular basement membrane. Clinical Nephrology. 1977;**7**:65-72

[9] Fervenza FC, Sethi S, Glassock RJ. Idiopathic membranoproliferative glomerulonephritis: Does it exist? Nephrology, Dialysis, Transplantation. 2012;**27**:4288-4294

[10] Burkholder PM, Marchand A, Krueger RP. Mixed membranous and proliferative glomerulonephritis. A correlative light, immunofluorescence, and electron microscopic study. Laboratory Investigation. 1970;**23**:459-479

[11] Berger J, Galle P. Dense deposits within the basal membranes of the kidney. Optical and electron microscopic study. Presse Médicale. 1963;**71**:2351-2354

[12] Habib R, Kleinknecht C, Gubler MC, Levy M. Idiopathic membranoproliferative glomerulonephritis in children. Report of 105 cases. Clinical Nephrology. 1973;**1**:194-214

[13] D'Agati VD, Bomback AS. C3 glomerulopathy: What's in a name? Kidney International. 2012;**82**:379-381

[14] Appel GB, Cook HT, Hageman G, Jennette JC, Kashgarian M, Kirschfink M, et al. Membranoproliferative glomerulonephritis type II (dense deposit disease): An update. Journal of the American Society of Nephrology. 2005;**16**:1392-1403

[15] Roccatello D, Fornasieri A, Giachino O, Rossi D, Beltrame A, Banfi G, et al. Multicenter study on hepatitis C virus-related cryoglobulinemic glomerulonephritis. American Journal of Kidney Diseases. 2007;**49**:69-82

[16] Smith KD, Alpers CE. Pathogenic mechanisms in membranoproliferative glomerulonephritis. Current Opinion in Nephrology and Hypertension. 2005;**14**:396-403

[17] Strife CF, McAdams AJ, McEnery PT, Bove KE, West CD. Hypocomplementemic and normocomplementemic acute nephritis in children: A comparison with respect to etiology, clinical manifestations, and glomerular morphology. The Journal of Pediatrics. 1974;**84**:29-38

[18] Joh K, Aizawa S, Matsuyama N, Yamaguchi Y, Kitajima T, Sakai O, et al. Morphologic variations of dense deposit disease: Light and electron microscopic, immunohistochemical and clinical findings in 10 patients. Acta Pathol Jpn. 1993;**43**:552-565

[19] Walker PD. Dense deposit disease: New insights. Current Opinion in Nephrology and Hypertension. 2007;**16**:204-212

[20] Walker PD, Ferrario F, Joh K, Bonsib SM. Dense deposit disease is not a membranoproliferative glomerulonephritis. Modern Pathology. 2007;**20**:605-616

[21] Sethi S, Fervenza FC, Zhang Y, Zand L, Meyer NC, Borsa N, et al. Atypical postinfectious glomerulonephritis is associated with abnormalities in the alternative pathway of complement. Kidney International. 2013;**83**:293-299

[22] Hou J, Markowitz GS, Bomback AS, Appel GB, Herlitz LC, Barry Stokes M, et al. Toward a working definition of C3 glomerulopathy by immunofluorescence. Kidney International. 2014;**85**:450-456

[23] Levy M, Gubler MC, Sich M, Beziau A, Habib R. Immunopathology of membranoproliferative glomerulonephritis with subendothelial deposits (Type I MPGN). Clinical Immunology and Immunopathology. 1978;**10**:477-492

[24] Sethi S, Fervenza FC, Zhang Y, Zand L, Vrana JA, Nasr SH, et al. C3 glomerulonephritis: Clinicopathological findings, complement abnormalities, glomerular proteomic profile, treatment, and follow-up. Kidney International. 2012;**82**:465-473

[25] Sethi S, Gamez JD, Vrana JA, Theis JD, Bergen HR, Zipfel PF, et al. Glomeruli of dense deposit disease contain components of the alternative and terminal complement pathway. Kidney International. 2009;**75**:952-960

[26] Zhang Y, Meyer NC, Wang K, Nishimura C, Frees K, Jones M, et al. Causes of alternative pathway dysregulation in dense deposit disease. Clinical Journal of the American Society of Nephrology. 2012;**7**:265-274

[27] Fakhouri F, Frémeaux-Bacchi V, Noël LH, Cook HT, Pickering MC. C3 glomerulopathy: A new classification. Nature Reviews. Nephrology. 2010;**6**:494-499

[28] Larsen CP, Walker PD. Redefining C3 glomerulopathy: 'C3 only' is a bridge too far. Kidney International. 2013;**83**:331-332

[29] Sethi S, Nester CM, Smith RJ. Membranoproliferative glomerulonephritis and C3 glomerulopathy: Resolving the confusion. Kidney International. 2012;**81**:434-441

[30] Pickering M, Cook HT. Complement and glomerular disease: New insights. Current Opinion in Nephrology and Hypertension. 2011;**20**:271-277

[31] Pickering MC, D'Agati VD, Nester CM, Smith RJ, Haas M, Appel GB, et al. C3 glomerulopathy: Consensus report. Kidney International. 2013;**84**:1079-1089

[32] Cook H, Pickering M. C3 glomerulopathies, including dense deposit disease. In: Jennete J, Olson J, Silva F, D'Agati V, editors. Heptinstall's Pathology of the Kidney. Philadelphia: Wolters Kluwer; 2015. pp. 341-366

[33] Cook HT. Evolving complexity of complement-related diseases: C3 glomerulopathy and atypical haemolytic uremic syndrome. Current Opinion in Nephrology and Hypertension. 2018;**27**:165-170

[34] Sibley RK, Kim Y. Dense intramembranous deposit disease: New pathologic features. Kidney International. 1984;**25**:660-670

[35] Schwertz R, Rother U, Anders D, Gretz N, Schärer K, Kirschfink M. Complement analysis in children with idiopathic membranoproliferative glomerulonephritis: A long-term follow-up. Pediatric Allergy and Immunology. 2001;**12**:166-172

[36] Lu DF, Moon M, Lanning LD, McCarthy AM, Smith RJ. Clinical features and outcomes of 98 children and adults with dense deposit disease. Pediatric Nephrology. 2012;**27**:773-781

[37] Walport MJ, Davies KA, Botto M, Naughton MA, Isenberg DA, Biasi D, et al. C3 nephritic factor and SLE: Report of four cases and review of the literature. QJM. 1994;**87**:609-615

[38] Sheeran TP, White RH, Raafat F, Jackson MA, Kumararatne DS, Situnayake RD. Hypocomplementaemia, C3 nephritic factor and type III mesangiocapillary glomerulonephritis progressing to systemic lupus erythematosus. British Journal of Rheumatology. 1995;**34**:90-92

[39] Cronin CC, Higgins TJ, Molloy M. Lupus, C3 nephritic factor and partial lipodystrophy. QJM. 1995;**88**:298-299

[40] Frémeaux-Bacchi V, Weiss L, Demouchy C, May A, Palomera S, Kazatchkine MD. Hypocomplementaemia of poststreptococcal acute glomerulonephritis is associated with C3 nephritic factor (C3NeF) IgG autoantibody activity. Nephrology, Dialysis, Transplantation. 1994;**9**:1747-1750

[41] Hageman GS, Hancox LS, Taiber AJ, Gehrs KM, Anderson DH, Johnson LV, et al. Extended haplotypes in the complement factor H (CFH) and CFH-related (CFHR) family of genes protect against age-related macular degeneration: Characterization, ethnic distribution and evolutionary implications. Annals of Medicine. 2006;**38**:592-604

[42] Colville D, Guymer R, Sinclair RA, Savige J. Visual impairment caused by retinal abnormalities in mesangiocapillary (membranoproliferative) glomerulonephritis type II ("dense deposit disease"). American Journal of Kidney Diseases. 2003;**42**:E2-E5

[43] Holz FG, Pauleikhoff D, Klein R, Bird AC. Pathogenesis of lesions in late age-related macular disease. American Journal of Ophthalmology. 2004;**137**:504-510

[44] Abrera-Abeleda MA, Nishimura C, Smith JL, Sethi S, McRae JL, Murphy BF, et al. Variations in the complement regulatory genes factor H (CFH) and factor H related 5 (CFHR5) are associated with membranoproliferative glomerulonephritis type II (dense deposit disease). Journal of Medical Genetics. 2006;**43**:582-589

[45] Misra A, Peethambaram A, Garg A. Clinical features and metabolic and autoimmune derangements in acquired partial lipodystrophy: Report of 35 cases and review of the literature. Medicine (Baltimore). 2004;**83**:18-34

[46] Ormos J, Mágori A, Sonkodi S, Streitmann K. Type 2 membranoproliferative glomerulonephritis with electron-dense basement membrane alteration in the spleen. Archives of Pathology & Laboratory Medicine. 1979;**103**:265-266

[47] Thorner P, Baumal R. Extraglomerular dense deposits in dense deposit disease. Archives of Pathology & Laboratory Medicine. 1982;**106**:628-631

[48] Weidner N, Lorentz WB. Three-dimensional studies of acellular glomerular basement membranes in dense-deposit disease. Virchows Archiv. A, Pathological Anatomy and Histopathology. 1986;**409**:595-607

[49] Gale DP, de Jorge EG, Cook HT, Martinez-Barricarte R, Hadjisavvas A, McLean AG, et al. Identification of a mutation in complement factor H-related protein 5 in patients of Cypriot origin with glomerulonephritis. Lancet. 2010;**376**:794-801

[50] Malik TH, Lavin PJ, Goicoechea de Jorge E, Vernon KA, Rose KL, Patel MP, et al. A hybrid CFHR3-1 gene causes familial C3 glomerulopathy. Journal of the American Society of Nephrology. 2012;**23**:1155-1160

[51] Medjeral-Thomas NR, O'Shaughnessy MM, O'Regan JA, Traynor C, Flanagan M, Wong L, et al. C3 glomerulopathy: Clinicopathologic features and predictors of outcome. Clinical Journal of the American Society of Nephrology. 2014;**9**:46-53

[52] Okuda Y, Ishikura K, Hamada R, Harada R, Sakai T, Hamasaki Y, et al. Membrano-proliferative glomerulonephritis and C3 glomerulonephritis: Frequency, clinical features, and outcome in children. Nephrology (Carlton). 2015;**20**:286-292

[53] Kersnik Levart T, Ferluga D, Vizjak A, Mraz J, Kojc N. Severe active C3 glomerulonephritis triggered by immune complexes and inactivated after eculizumab therapy. Diagnostic Pathology. 2016;**11**:94

[54] Berger SP, Roos A, Daha MR. Complement and the kidney: What the nephrologist needs to know in 2006? Nephrology, Dialysis, Transplantation. 2005;**20**:2613-2619

[55] Thurman JM, Holers VM. The central role of the alternative complement pathway in human disease. Journal of Immunology. 2006;**176**:1305-1310

[56] Zipfel PF, Smith RJ, Skerka C. Factor I and factor H deficiency in renal diseases: Similar defects in the fluid phase have a different outcome at the surface of the glomerular basement membrane. Nephrology, Dialysis, Transplantation. 2009;**24**:385-387

[57] Vernon KA, Ruseva MM, Cook HT, Botto M, Malik TH, Pickering MC. Partial complement factor H deficiency associates with C3 glomerulopathy and thrombotic microangiopathy. Journal of the American Society of Nephrology. 2016;**27**:1334-1342

[58] Gharavi AG, Kiryluk K, Choi M, Li Y, Hou P, Xie J, et al. Genome-wide association study identifies susceptibility loci for IgA nephropathy. Nature Genetics. 2011;**43**:321-327

[59] Hughes AE, Orr N, Esfandiary H, Diaz-Torres M, Goodship T, Chakravarthy U. A common CFH haplotype, with deletion of CFHR1 and CFHR3, is associated with lower risk of age-related macular degeneration. Nature Genetics. 2006;**38**:1173-1177

[60] Hebecker M, Józsi M. Factor H-related protein 4 activates complement by serving as a platform for the assembly of alternative pathway C3 convertase via its interaction with C3b protein. The Journal of Biological Chemistry. 2012;**287**:19528-19536

[61] Skerka C, Chen Q, Fremeaux-Bacchi V, Roumenina LT. Complement factor H related proteins (CFHRs). Molecular Immunology. 2013;**56**:170-180

[62] Goicoechea de Jorge E, Caesar JJ, Malik TH, Patel M, Colledge M, Johnson S, et al. Dimerization of complement factor H-related proteins modulates complement activation in vivo. Proceedings of the National Academy of Sciences of the United States of America. 2013;**110**:4685-4690

[63] Medjeral-Thomas NR, Lomax-Browne HJ, Beckwith H, Willicombe M, McLean AG, Brookes P, et al. Circulating complement factor H-related proteins 1 and 5 correlate with disease activity in IgA nephropathy. Kidney International. 2017;**92**:942-952

[64] Athanasiou Y, Voskarides K, Gale DP, Damianou L, Patsias C, Zavros M, et al. Familial C3 glomerulopathy associated with CFHR5 mutations: Clinical characteristics of 91 patients in 16 pedigrees. Clinical Journal of the American Society of Nephrology. 2011; **6**:1436-1446

[65] Medjeral-Thomas N, Malik TH, Patel MP, Toth T, Cook HT, Tomson C, et al. A novel CFHR5 fusion protein causes C3 glomerulopathy in a family without Cypriot ancestry. Kidney International. 2014;**85**:933-937

[66] Tortajada A, Yébenes H, Abarrategui-Garrido C, Anter J, García-Fernández JM, Martínez-Barricarte R, et al. C3 glomerulopathy-associated CFHR1 mutation alters FHR oligomerization and complement regulation. The Journal of Clinical Investigation. 2013;**123**:2434-2446

[67] Wong EKS, Kavanagh D. Diseases of complement dysregulation—An overview. Seminars in Immunopathology. 2018;**40**:49-64

[68] Zhao W, Ding Y, Lu J, Zhang T, Chen D, Zhang H, et al. Genetic analysis of the complement pathway in C3 glomerulopathy. Nephrology, Dialysis, Transplantation. 2018:1-9. DOI: 10.1093/ndt/gfy033

[69] Martínez-Barricarte R, Heurich M, Valdes-Cañedo F, Vazquez-Martul E, Torreira E, Montes T, et al. Human C3 mutation reveals a mechanism of dense deposit disease pathogenesis and provides insights into complement activation and regulation. The Journal of Clinical Investigation. 2010;**120**:3702-3712

[70] Servais A, Noël LH, Dragon-Durey MA, Gübler MC, Rémy P, Buob D, et al. Heterogeneous pattern of renal disease associated with homozygous factor H deficiency. Human Pathology. 2011;**42**:1305-1311

[71] Tarshish P, Bernstein J, Tobin JN, Edelmann CM. Treatment of mesangiocapillary glomerulonephritis with alternate-day prednisone—A report of the International Study of Kidney Disease in Children. Pediatric Nephrology. 1992;**6**:123-130

[72] Rudnicki M. Rituximab for Treatment of Membranoproliferative Glomerulonephritis and C3 Glomerulopathies. BioMed Research International. 2017;**2017**:2180508

[73] Giaime P, Daniel L, Burtey S. Remission of C3 glomerulopathy with rituximab as only immunosuppressive therapy. Clinical Nephrology. 2015;**83**:57-60

[74] Daina E, Noris M, Remuzzi G. Eculizumab in a patient with dense-deposit disease. The New England Journal of Medicine. 2012;**366**:1161-1163

[75] Nester CM, Brophy PD. Eculizumab in the treatment of atypical haemolytic uraemic syndrome and other complement-mediated renal diseases. Current Opinion in Pediatrics. 2013;**25**:225-231

[76] Herlitz LC, Bomback AS, Markowitz GS, Stokes MB, Smith RN, Colvin RB, et al. Pathology after eculizumab in dense deposit disease and C3 GN. Journal of the American Society of Nephrology. 2012;**23**:1229-1237

4

Chronic Kidney Disease and Coronary Artery Disease

Eduardo Gomes Lima, Daniel Valente Batista,
Eduardo Bello Martins and Whady Hueb

Abstract

Chronic kidney disease (CKD) and coronary artery disease (CAD) are conditions that, when present together, is considered a high-risk feature. Despite the high prevalence, few studies are dedicated to studying CAD specifically in individuals with CKD, and it is a common exclusion criterion in most trials. This fact leads to gap in the evidence for the management of CAD, which, sometimes, results in undertreatment of CKD patients. In this chapter, authors present peculiarities related to CAD among patients with CKD from physiopathology to diagnostic and therapeutic decisions. An evidence-based approach was used to explore this high-risk subset of CAD patients.

Keywords: chronic kidney disease, coronary artery disease, atherosclerosis, coronary artery bypass graft, percutaneous coronary intervention

1. Background

The association between chronic kidney disease (CKD) and coronary artery disease (CAD) has been the subject of numerous studies recently. Not only because of the frequent association between the two entities, but also because of the aggregate risk when both conditions are present in the same individual.

Despite the high prevalence, few studies are dedicated to studying CAD specifically in individuals with CKD. In fact, CKD, especially in its final stages, is a common exclusion criterion in large studies. This fact resulted in a gap in the evidence for the management of CAD, which, sometimes, results in undertreatment of CKD patients.

This chapter aims to explore the association between CAD and CKD, approaching from pathophysiology to available evidence for the treatment of these conditions.

2. Coronary atherosclerosis and renal failure

Another scenario where there is a profound interaction between renal failure and the cardiovascular system is with regard to coronary atherosclerosis. It is known that chronic kidney disease adds risk to coronary events. The relationship between renal disease and cardiovascular mortality can be found even in the early stages of disease [1] and increases as kidney function deteriorates [2] (see **Table 1** for the stages of CKD according to the National Kidney Foundation KDOQI Clinical Practice Guidelines [3]). It is also known that the population with CAD and CKD has higher mortality regardless of the treatment used for coronary disease [4].

Several epidemiological studies have demonstrated that CKD is an independent risk factor for cardiovascular events.

The Framingham Heart Study was one of the first to associate chronic kidney disease with cardiovascular events in the general population. Of the 6233 study participants, stage 2 CKD was found in 246 men and 270 women. Of these, 81% were not diagnosed with cardiovascular disease at the start of the study. After 15 years of follow-up, there was a tendency for a higher incidence of cardiovascular events in the male population with stage 2 CKD [5]. Data from the Atherosclerosis Risk in the Communities study also confirm an increase in the risk of cardiovascular events in this same population [6]. When GFR is considered as a continuous variable, this study points to a 5–6% increase in cardiovascular risk for each loss of 10 mL/min/1.73 m^2 of GFR. Go and colleagues also demonstrated, in a cohort study of 1,120,295 patients, comprised of approximately 9.6% of diabetics and 6.3% of CAD patients, a risk of death of about 1.2 times higher associated with an GFR 45–59 mL/min/1.73 m^2 when compared to those with GFR ≥60 mL/min/1.73 m^2 [7]. There was a growing risk as the lowest GFR was considered, culminating with a relative risk of about 5.9 in those patients with RFG <15 mL/min/1.73 m^2.

There is also a worse prognosis associated with renal failure in populations with established heart disease. The Valsartan in Acute Myocardial Infarction Trial (VALIANT) looks at the influence of GFR, even in its early stages, in a population at high risk for cardiovascular

Stages	GFR (mL/min/1.73 m^2)	CKD
0	>90	Risk group for CKD. Absence of renal injury
1	>90	Normal renal function. Presence of kidney damage
2	89–60	Discrete or functional CKD
3	59–30	Moderate or laboratory CKD
4	29–15	Severe or clinical CKD
5	<15	Terminal or pre-dialytic CKD

Table 1. Staging and classification of CKD.

events [8]. This study accompanied patients after acute myocardial infarction complicated by systolic ventricular dysfunction or symptoms of congestive heart failure (CHF) who were randomized to either valsartan, captopril or both. After adjusting for the received treatment and comorbidities, a risk of 1.14 times greater risk for cardiovascular death was found in patients with an GFR of 60–74 mL/min/1.73 m^2 (95% CI 1.02–1.27) and 1.10 times for combined events (cardiac mortality, re-infarction, CHF and stroke) when compared to the population with normal renal function. A factor that may have contributed to these findings is that the CKD population was undertreated when compared to the population with normal renal function, receiving invasive stratification (27.5% vs. 34.7%) and beta-blockers (71.9% vs. 74.7%) to a lesser extent than those with preserved renal function.

2.1. Mechanisms of cardiovascular complications in CKD

As previously described, kidney disease, even in its early stages, poses an increased risk of cardiovascular events. Even initial lesions such as a discrete fall in GFR or microalbuminuria (including patients with normal GFR) are associated with increased cardiac mortality, AMI or stroke. The main pathophysiological mechanism involved in this complex relationship appears to be endothelial dysfunction.

2.1.1. Endothelial dysfunction

Endothelial dysfunction is one of the initial events of the so-called atherosclerotic gait. It is present in both small and large vessels. Reducing the bioavailability of nitric oxide (NO) is one of the main mechanisms involved in endothelial dysfunction in patients with GFR. In this context, it is important to highlight the role of asymmetric dimethyl arginine (ADMA), which is derived from protein catabolism and competitive inhibitor of NO synthase produced mainly in the endothelium, the heart and the smooth cells and is clarified by the kidneys. When in high concentrations, as in individuals with GFR, it blocks the entry of L-arginine at the cellular level, leading to a reduction in NO synthesis. This leads to increased peripheral vascular resistance, intimal hyperplasia of the vessels and consequent increase in blood pressure with remodeling of the same. Recent studies have pointed to ADMA as an independent marker of cardiovascular risk in individuals with CAD [9].

2.1.2. Albuminuria

The correlation between macroalbuminuria and microalbuminuria with endothelial dysfunction measured in peripheral vessels is something that has been demonstrated and is a consequence of glomerular hyperfiltration. Thus, albuminuria has been identified not only as a consequence of the renal aggression that precedes the fall of GFR, but also as powerful marker of cardiovascular risk. Like GFR, albuminuria increases cardiovascular risk even at minimal levels. This risk increases as the albuminuria level rises, defined as normal albumin excretion (<30 mg/g), to microalbuminuria (30–300 mg/g) and, finally, with macroalbuminuria (>300 mg/g).

Several studies have demonstrated the role of albuminuria as a marker of cardiovascular risk. The Irbesartan Diabetic Nephropathy Trial (IDNT) studied 1715 subjects with type 2 DM, hypertension and macroalbuminuria, randomizing them to receive irbesartan, amlodipine or placebo. In a post-hoc analysis of Anavekar [10], univariate analysis showed an increase in cardiovascular risk proportional to the value of albuminuria. Multivariate analysis confirmed albuminuria as an independent risk factor. The (Reduction of End Points in NIDDM with Angiotensin II Antagonist Losartan (RENAAL) study [11] showed similar results, demonstrating a 1.92-fold higher risk of cardiovascular events in the group with albuminuria >3000 mg/g when compared to the dose group <1500 mg/g. The HOPE [12] study got a RR of 1.83 for cardiac death and 1.61 for the combined outcome of AMI or stroke in the population with albuminuria >17.7 mg/g. In addition, subsequent analyzes of HOPE suggest that albuminuria as low as 4.4 mg/g already translates into increased cardiovascular risk, suggesting that it behaves as a continuous variable [13].

2.1.3. Systemic arterial hypertension

Hypertension is present in most patients with CKD and atherosclerotic disease. The activation of the renin-angiotensin-aldosterone system (RAAS), sympathetic nervous system and sodium retention plays an important role in the development of hypertension. Recently, renalase, a regulator of cardiac function and blood pressure produced by the kidney, has been discovered. This regulator metabolizes catecholamines and has hypotensive action. Its absence may be responsible for adrenergic hyperreactivity leading to endothelial dysfunction and cardiac and vascular remodeling [9].

The activation of RAAS occurs in several ways in kidney disease. Angiotensin II stimulates NAD (P) H oxidase, leading to superoxide anion formation and contributing to endothelial dysfunction and cardiac remodeling. In addition, when angiotensin II stimulates the AT 1 receptor, there is generation of reactive oxygen species (ROS) with release of inflammatory mediators, including cytokines, adhesion molecules, PAI-1 (plasminogen activator inhibitor-1), among others. These events eventually promote the progression of atherosclerosis.

2.1.4. Inflammation

Atherosclerosis has been considered as an inflammatory condition. CKD patients are known as 'inflamed patients' since we have evidence of measurable inflammatory markers such as C-reactive protein (CRP), fibrinogen, interleukin-6 (IL-6), tumor necrosis factor-alpha (TNF-alpha), factor VIIc, factor VIIIc, plasmin-antiplasmin complex, D-dimer, E-selectin, VCAM-1 and ICAM1, as well as the deleterious effects of the inflammatory process in this population [9]. The poor nutrition of these patients, evidenced by low levels of albumin, pre-albumin and transferrin, has been suggested as a possible mechanism of activation of the inflammatory process. In addition, oxidative stress, the accumulation of modified molecules after synthesis, nonenzymatic glycosylation products or other products normally cleansed by the kidney also have their role in triggering inflammation [9]. Consequently, we have alterations in the endothelium and lipoproteins leading to accelerated atherosclerosis.

CRP has been particularly studied in the chronic kidney population, being found at higher levels in the terminal CKD population than in the normal population. CRP has been shown to be an excellent marker of cardiovascular risk in this population [14, 15].

The inflammation also seems to be related to the vascular calcification process, so common in patients with CKD, markedly in those in advanced stages of the disease. Calcification may be present in the medial layer of vessels, smooth muscle cells, medial muscular arteries and valvular system. As calcification progress, the capacitance of the arterial vessels is reduced, promoting the progression of systemic arterial hypertension (SAH) and left ventricular hypertrophy (LVH). The mechanisms involved in the CKD calcification process are complex and include the passive precipitation of Ca and P in the presence of high concentrations of these ions in the extracellular, in addition to the effect of inducers of osteogenic transformation, formation of hydroxyapatite and deficiency of calcification inhibitors such as osteoprotegerin and fetuin-A. In addition, high levels of leptin, common in patients with CKD due to reduced GFR, can induce calcification via hypothalamic receptors, stimulating osteoblastic beta-adrenergic receptors, generating ROS and inducing bone morphogenetic protein-2 (BMP-2). BMPs are regulators of bone formation, acting on receptors (BMPRs) that modulate gene expression. BMP-2 and BMP-4 are promoters of calcification, while BMP-7 behaves as an inhibitor of this process. BMP-7 is expressed mainly in the kidney and its reduction is proportional to the loss of renal function (**Figure 1**) [9].

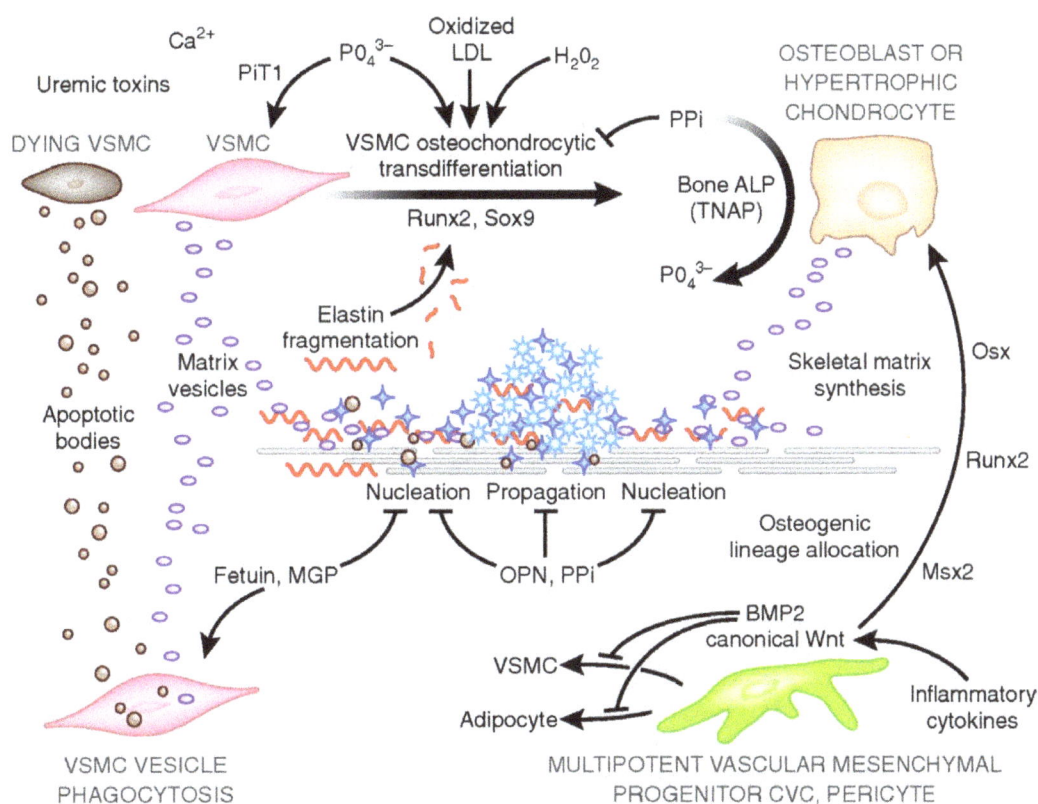

Figure 1. Atherosclerosis and calcification in renal failure. Extracted from Mizobuchi et al. [35].

3. Particularities in the diagnosis and treatment of CAD in patients with renal insufficiency

The incidence of coronary disease in the CKD population is high. Gowdak and colleagues observed a 47% incidence of angiographically significant CAD among patients with terminal CKD awaiting renal transplantation [16]. Interestingly, even in the population without traditional risk factors (SAH, DM, obesity, dyslipidemia and smoking), the observed incidence of CAD was 26%, and may reach 100% among those with all risk factors mentioned above.

The best method to investigate or stratify CAD in this population is still a matter of dispute. The presence of endothelial dysfunction, LVH, hypertension and volume overload in chronic renal patients should be considered when choosing the best method.

Some studies have considered that a more aggressive strategy should be used, since the non-invasive methods do not have good accuracy in the prediction of events in this population, especially in those with terminal CKD. In an attempt to validate a strategy for diagnosis of significant CAD in a population of chronic dialysis patients, a study conducted at the Heart Institute of the Hospital das Clínicas of the USP Medical School (InCor-HCFMUSP) confirms that the documented coronary angiography and the presence of DM were good predictors of cardiovascular events. The sensitivity, specificity and positive and negative predictive values of myocardial scintigraphy with dipyridamole were 70, 74, 69 and 71%, respectively. It is worth noting that scintigraphy did not diagnose CAD in a significant number of patients with CAD confirmed by coronary angiography [16, 17]. These data confirm that the invasive strategy remains the gold standard in the diagnosis and stratification of risk in this population. It is important to remember that the use of iodinated contrast (especially in the population with discrete to moderate CRF) may worsen the renal function of these individuals, and the need for hemodialysis in cases of contrast-induced nephropathy is not uncommon. This, in addition to being an invasive, more expensive and less available method, does not authorize us to indicate routine coronary angiography for patients with CKD in the investigation and/or stratification of CAD. Clinical judgment should weigh the risk factors already mentioned to select the population that will benefit most from the invasive examination.

The use of new methods for the diagnosis of CAD, such as coronary angiotomography, calcium score and magnetic resonance imaging has also been studied in this population. In a recently published study, the calcium score applied to a population of renal transplant candidates had a good correlation with angiographic CAD for diagnosis, as well as being a good predictor of cardiovascular events when above 400 Agatston [18]. Magnetic resonance imaging has its importance mainly in the evaluation of previous infarctions, ischemia and myocardial viability in this population [19].

4. Treatment of CAD in patients with CKD

Treatment of coronary disease is based on optimized medical therapy associated or not with interventional procedures (surgical revascularization or angioplasty). The population with CAD and CKD has peculiarities that should not be forgotten when choosing the best therapeutic strategy.

The population of chronic renal failure with CAD is certainly a subgroup that benefits as much as possible from full clinical management because it is a group of patients with multiple comorbidities and an accelerated atherosclerosis [20]. In spite of this recommendation, the population with renal dysfunction is frequently undertreated, which surely contributes to the worse prognosis of this special population [21].

Interventional therapy in patients with chronic kidney disease with CAD seems to be beneficial in some situations, especially when we consider their high atherosclerotic load and angiographic complexity.

A retrospective study by Reddan, conducted at Duke University, analyzed 4584 patients with CAD who underwent clinical treatment, percutaneous coronary intervention (PCI) or myocardial revascularization (CABG), who were stratified according to GFR, followed and evaluated for cardiovascular events. In this study, a benefit of percutaneous treatment over clinical treatment was observed in the population with mild to moderate CRF, but not among those with terminal CKD. When comparing myocardial revascularization surgery with medical treatment, we observed that, curiously, the benefit of surgery is greater as the severity of renal failure progresses [4].

In our setting stands out a subanalysis of MASS II [22], conducted by Lopes and collaborators at InCor - HCFMUSP. In this publication, 611 patients from the original study, randomized to medical treatment, PCI or CABG, were stratified by GFR in 3 categories (RFG > 90, between 89 and 60 or between 59 and 30 mL/min/1.73 m²) and classified as with normal renal function (n = 112/18%), mild (n = 349/57%) or moderate (n = 150/25%), respectively. The results point to a higher mortality among the population with moderate CRF, compared to the other two groups. In addition, it was observed that among patients with mild CRF, patients submitted to surgery had a higher survival rate free of cardiovascular events and lower mortality in 5 years compared to the population submitted to angioplasty or in exclusive medical treatment.

Lima and collaborators evaluated in a registry-type study 763 diabetic patients with CAD of the MASS group stratified according to renal function and followed for about 5 years. Of note is the high rate of CKD patients when applied clearance estimated by Cockcroft-Gault, with almost 65% of patients with some degree of CKD having clearance <90 mL/min. Even in an exclusively diabetic population, the presence of CKD was associated with higher mortality regardless of the treatment received, with survival rates of 91.1%, 89.6% and 76.2% for the preserved function, mild and moderate CKD, respectively (p = 0.001). When compared to the drug treatment, the surgical treatment was associated with lower combined event rates in the stratum with discrete CKD (86.2% versus 65.7% for CABG and TM respectively, p < 0.001) and additional revascularization in all function strata studied.

4.1. Interventional treatment in patients with end-stage CKD

This is a population where, despite the interventional therapy chosen, there is a higher risk of morbidity and mortality when compared to the general population. A patient undergoing CABG has a 4.4-fold greater risk of in-hospital death, a 3.1-fold increase in mediastinitis, and a 2.6-fold increase in stroke than a nondialysis patient. Some studies point to the safety of angioplasty in this population, especially in single-vessel patients [23]. However, when we compare angioplasty with surgical revascularization, it seems to bring greater cardiovascular protection to these patients [24]. This can be attributed to a higher rate of restenosis in this population, which is derived from a close association with diabetes mellitus, accelerated atherosclerosis and vascular calcification [25].

Several studies in chronic coronary disease have evaluated the performance of the subpopulation of chronic renal patients in their trials. In a post-hoc analysis of the ARTS study [26], 142 patients with moderate CKD with multiarterial CAD were randomized to receive surgery or angioplasty and followed for 5 years. Regardless of the revascularization method chosen, patients with moderate CRF had more cardiovascular events (death, stroke, nonfatal AMI or additional revascularization) than the population with mild or normal renal function. When we compared the strategies, we observed that there was no significant difference in mortality (RR: 1.18, 95% CI: 0.51–2.72, p = 0.81), but a greater number of events combined in the angioplasty group (RR: 1.56, 95% CI: 1.03–2.37, p = 0.04), mainly due to additional revascularizations (29% vs. 9.6% p = 0.005).

The BARI study [27] evaluated 3608 patients (randomized and from the registry), stratifying them into two groups: with and without CRF, which was defined as baseline serum creatinine greater than 1.5 mg/dL. Of the total, 1517 patients were submitted to surgery and 2091 to angioplasty. Of these, 76 patients were considered to have chronic renal failure. This population was older and had a higher proportion of hypertensive and diabetic patients. Among patients undergoing PCI, chronic kidney disease had a higher incidence of in-hospital mortality and cardiogenic shock. In addition, this population was more susceptible to the presence of angina, hospitalizations due to cardiac reasons and less time for additional revascularization compared to the normal population. In 7 years, the population with CKD had a higher incidence of general (RR: 2.2, p < 0.001) and heart (RR: 2.8, p < 0.001) than the population with normal renal function.

Although we consider the benefit of pharmacological stents on conventional stents with regard to the lower incidence of restenosis, recent studies comparing pharmacological stents with CABG in this population show a greater benefit of the latter, especially at the expense of lower rate of additional revascularization [28]. A recent study by Marui and colleagues from the CREDO-Kyoto registry demonstrated that in 388 patients with dialytic CKD, similar incidences of general and cardiac death were observed when CABG compared with PCI in a long-term follow-up. The latter strategy, however, was associated with higher rates of AMI and additional revascularization [29].

In the post-hoc analysis of the FREEDOM study [30], comparison of interventional strategies among diabetic patients with CAD in the presence of renal dysfunction defined by estimated clearance <60 mL/min did not demonstrate superiority of CABG on PCI with first-generation pharmacological stent at MACCE rate at 5-year follow-up.

Charytan et al. [31] in a collaborative study including 10 randomized prospective studies of 3993 subjects demonstrated similar survival rates at 5 years when patients with CKD class 3–5 underwent CABG or PCI (HR 0.99, CI 0.67–1.46). However, AMI-free survival among patients with CKD class 3–5 was higher among those undergoing surgical treatment (HR: 0.49; CI: 0.29–0.82). Consistent with other studies, CABG was associated with lower rates of additional revascularization than PCI, regardless of the renal function stratum considered.

Recently, a meta-analysis by Bundhun's et al. [32] included 18 studies involving a larger number of patients (n = 69,456, 29,239 underwent CABG and 40,217 underwent PCI). This present analysis observed a benefit of CABG in reducing mortality when compared to PCI in long-term follow-up only (OR: 0.81, 95% CI: 0.70–0.94, p = 0.007 for nondialytic, OR: 0.81, 95% CI: 0.69–096, P = 0.01 for dialytic). It is also worth mentioning a benefit in reducing additional revascularizations among those submitted to CABG in almost all studies that included this outcome. Of note, however, is the heterogeneity of the included studies, with different definitions for CKD, in addition to follow-up times ranging from 1 month to 8 years.

Off-pump CABG was also evaluated in some studies because of the theoretical benefit of a less aggressive procedure than on-pump CABG. These studies have demonstrated a lower need for blood products and dialysis in the postoperative period, shorter hospital stay in intensive care and mechanical ventilation, but with no difference in mortality in the medium term [24, 33]. Consistent with these previous results, recently published data from the Coronary Artery Bypass Grafting Surgery Off-pump Revascularization Study, comparing on-pump versus off-pump CABG, showed a reduced risk of perioperative acute renal injury associated with off-pump CABG. In spite of this, no renal protection was observed at the 1-year follow-up associated with this surgical strategy [34].

5. Final considerations

CKD has a negative impact on the prognosis of individuals with CAD regardless of the treatment. There are no peculiarities in the indication of revascularization in this population, and attention must be paid to the greater clinical and angiographic severity of this population. The drug treatment should be applied considering the potential limitations of the use of some classes among those with terminal CKD, however, avoiding at all costs under-treatment. There is still no consensus on the best therapeutic strategy for CAD (e.g. interventional versus conservative; PCI versus CABG) for those with CKD. The studies are heterogeneous and almost completeness formed by observational records, post-hoc analyses of large trials or meta-analyses. In spite of this, some clarity seems to emerge from these publications: (1) the greater the angiographic severity/severity of CKD, the greater is the benefit of surgical revascularization; (2) in the subpopulations with discrete/moderate CKD, there is no clear evidence of surgery on the other treatments; and (3) surgery is associated with less need for additional revascularization independently of the status of renal function, which suggests that this benefit is associated with the revascularization method itself, rather than the patient's renal status.

We await the results of the ISCHEMIA-CKD study (ClinicalTrials.gov Identifier: NCT01985360), designed to study patients with documented (at least moderate) ischemia and severe renal dysfunction (GFR <30 or on dialysis) randomized to an initial strategy of coronary angiography and interventional treatment plus optical medical therapy or optimal medical therapy alone. Its results will surely bring answers to pertinent questions not yet answered in this common clinical scenario.

Author details

Eduardo Gomes Lima*, Daniel Valente Batista, Eduardo Bello Martins and Whady Hueb

*Address all correspondence to: eduglima@yahoo.com.br

Department of Clinical Cardiology, Heart Institute (InCor), University of São Paulo, São Paulo, Brazil

References

[1] Polonsky TS, Locatelli F. The contribution of early nephropathy to cardiovascular risk. Cardiology Clinics. 2010;**28**:427-436

[2] Parikh NI, Hwang SJ, Larson MG, Levy D, Fox CS. Chronic kidney disease as a predictor of cardiovascular disease (from the Framingham Heart Study). The American Journal of Cardiology. 2008;**102**:47-53

[3] Levey AS, Coresh J, Balk E, et al. National Kidney Foundation practice guidelines for chronic kidney disease: Evaluation, classification, and stratification. Annals of Internal Medicine. 2003;**139**:137-147

[4] Reddan DN, Szczech LA, Tuttle RH, et al. Chronic kidney disease, mortality, and treatment strategies among patients with clinically significant coronary artery disease. Journal of the American Society of Nephrology. 2003;**14**:2373-2380

[5] Culleton BF, Larson MG, Wilson PW, Evans JC, Parfrey PS, Levy D. Cardiovascular disease and mortality in a community-based cohort with mild renal insufficiency. Kidney International. 1999;**56**:2214-2219

[6] Manjunath G, Tighiouart H, Ibrahim H, et al. Level of kidney function as a risk factor for atherosclerotic cardiovascular outcomes in the community. Journal of the American College of Cardiology. 2003;**41**:47-55

[7] Go AS, Chertow GM, Fan D, McCulloch CE, Hsu CY. Chronic kidney disease and the risks of death, cardiovascular events, and hospitalization. The New England Journal of Medicine. 2004;**351**:1296-1305

[8] Anavekar NS, McMurray JJ, Velazquez EJ, et al. Relation between renal dysfunction and cardiovascular outcomes after myocardial infarction. The New England Journal of Medicine. 2004;**351**:1285-1295

[9] Schiffrin EL, Lipman ML, Mann JF. Chronic kidney disease: Effects on the cardiovascular system. Circulation. 2007;**116**:85-97

[10] Anavekar NS, Gans DJ, Berl T, et al. Predictors of cardiovascular events in patients with type 2 diabetic nephropathy and hypertension: A case for albuminuria. Kidney International. 2004;**66**(Suppl 92):S50-S55

[11] Brenner BM, Cooper ME, de Zeeuw D, et al. Effects of losartan on renal and cardiovascular outcomes in patients with type 2 diabetes and nephropathy. The New England Journal of Medicine. 2001;**345**:861-869

[12] Heart Outcomes Prevention Evaluation Study Investigators. Effects of ramipril on cardiovascular and microvascular outcomes in people with diabetes mellitus: Results of the HOPE study and MICRO-HOPE substudy. Lancet. 2000;**355**:253-259

[13] Gerstein HC, Mann JF, Yi Q, et al. Albuminuria and risk of cardiovascular events, death, and heart failure in diabetic and nondiabetic individuals. JAMA. 2001;**286**:421-426

[14] Busch M, Franke S, Muller A, et al. Potential cardiovascular risk factors in chronic kidney disease: AGEs, total homocysteine and metabolites, and the C-reactive protein. Kidney International. 2004;**66**:338-347

[15] Menon V, Greene T, Wang X, et al. C-reactive protein and albumin as predictors of all-cause and cardiovascular mortality in chronic kidney disease. Kidney International. 2005;**68**:766-772

[16] Gowdak LH, de Paula FJ, Cesar LA, et al. Screening for significant coronary artery disease in high-risk renal transplant candidates. Coronary Artery Disease. 2007;**18**:553-558

[17] De Lima JJ, Wolff Gowdak LH, de Paula FJ, Ianhez LE, Franchini Ramires JA, Krieger EM. Validation of a strategy to diagnose coronary artery disease and predict cardiac events in high-risk renal transplant candidates. Coronary Artery Disease. 2010;**21**:164-167

[18] Rosario MA, Lima JJ, Parga JR, et al. Coronary calcium score as predictor of stenosis and events in pretransplant renal chronic failure. Arquivos Brasileiros de Cardiologia. 2010;**94**:236-243, 52-60, 9-47

[19] Andrade JM, Gowdak LH, Giorgi MC, et al. Cardiac MRI for detection of unrecognized myocardial infarction in patients with end-stage renal disease: Comparison with ECG and scintigraphy. American Journal of Roentgenology. 2009;**193**:W25-W32

[20] Montalescot G, Sechtem U, Achenbach S, et al. 2013 ESC guidelines on the management of stable coronary artery disease: The task force on the management of stable coronary artery disease of the European Society of Cardiology. European Heart Journal. 2013;**34**:2949-3003

[21] Berger AK, Duval S, Krumholz HM. Aspirin, beta-blocker, and angiotensin-converting enzyme inhibitor therapy in patients with end-stage renal disease and an acute myocardial infarction. Journal of the American College of Cardiology. 2003;**42**:201-208

[22] Lopes NH, da Silva Paulitsch F, Pereira A, et al. Mild chronic kidney dysfunction and treatment strategies for stable coronary artery disease. The Journal of Thoracic and Cardiovascular Surgery. 2009;**137**:1443-1449

[23] Reslerova M, Moe SM. Vascular calcification in dialysis patients: Pathogenesis and consequences. American Journal of Kidney Diseases. 2003;**41**:S96-S99

[24] Keeley EC, McCullough PA. Coronary revascularization in patients with end-stage renal disease: Risks, benefits, and optimal strategies. Reviews in Cardiovascular Medicine. 2003;**4**:125-130

[25] Ishio N, Kobayashi Y, Takebayashi H, et al. Impact of drug-eluting stents on clinical and angiographic outcomes in dialysis patients. Circulation Journal. 2007;**71**:1525-1529

[26] Aoki J, Ong AT, Hoye A, et al. Five year clinical effect of coronary stenting and coronary artery bypass grafting in renal insufficient patients with multivessel coronary artery disease: Insights from ARTS trial. European Heart Journal. 2005;**26**:1488-1493

[27] Szczech LA, Best PJ, Crowley E, et al. Outcomes of patients with chronic renal insufficiency in the bypass angioplasty revascularization investigation. Circulation. 2002;**105**:2253-2258

[28] Wang ZJ, Zhou YJ, Liu YY, et al. Comparison of drug-eluting stents and coronary artery bypass grafting for the treatment of multivessel coronary artery disease in patients with chronic kidney disease. Circulation Journal. 2009;**73**:1228-1234

[29] Marui A, Kimura T, Nishiwaki N, et al. Percutaneous coronary intervention versus coronary artery bypass grafting in patients with end-stage renal disease requiring dialysis (5-year outcomes of the CREDO-Kyoto PCI/CABG registry Cohort-2). The American Journal of Cardiology. 2014;**114**(4):555-561

[30] Baber U, Farkouh ME, Arbel Y, et al. Comparative efficacy of coronary artery bypass surgery vs. percutaneous coronary intervention in patients with diabetes and multivessel coronary artery disease with or without chronic kidney disease. European Heart Journal. 2016;**37**:3440-3447

[31] Charytan DM, Desai M, Mathur M, et al. Reduced risk of myocardial infarct and revascularization following coronary artery bypass grafting compared with percutaneous coronary intervention in patients with chronic kidney disease. Kidney International. 2016;**90**:411-421

[32] Bundhun PK, Bhurtu A, Chen MH. Impact of coronary artery bypass surgery and percutaneous coronary intervention on mortality in patients with chronic kidney disease and on dialysis: A systematic review and meta-analysis. Medicine (Baltimore). 2016;**95**:e4129

[33] Hage FG, Venkataraman R, Zoghbi GJ, Perry GJ, DeMattos AM, Iskandrian AE. The scope of coronary heart disease in patients with chronic kidney disease. Journal of the American College of Cardiology. 2009;**53**:2129-2140

[34] Garg AX, Devereaux PJ, Yusuf S, et al. Kidney function after off-pump or on-pump coronary artery bypass graft surgery: A randomized clinical trial. JAMA. 2014;**311**:2191-2198

[35] Mizobuchi et al. Vascular calcification: The killer of patients with chronic kidney disease. Journal of the American Society of Nephrology. 2009;**20**:1453-1464

5

Diabetic Nephropathy in Childhood: Predictive Tools and Preventive Strategies

Samuel N. Uwaezuoke, Ugo N. Chikani and
Ngozi R. Mbanefo

Abstract

Diabetic nephropathy is the commonest microvascular complication in both types 1 and 2 diabetes mellitus. Disease pathogenesis is based on a multifactorial interaction between metabolic and hemodynamic factors. In response to hyperglycemia, which disrupts the body's metabolic milieu, a cascade of complex molecular events occur leading to glomerular hypertrophy, tubular inflammation, mesangial expansion, oxidative stress, and renal fibrosis. Beyond the conventional microalbuminuria, which can predict disease onset, novel biomarkers are now proving more reliable as predictive tools. While several reports show that glomerular and tubular biomarkers are more sensitive than microalbuminuria, tubular markers specifically constitute earlier predictors of the disease. Similarly, biomarkers of inflammation and oxidative stress have been demonstrated as dependable diagnostic tools. As an important cause of mortality from end-stage renal disease (ESRD), diabetic nephropathy constitutes an important challenge in diabetic care. Interestingly, strict glycemic control assessed by glycated hemoglobin (Hb A1 c) estimates, and antihypertensive therapy with angiotensin-converting enzyme inhibitors/angiotensin-receptor blockers (ACEI/ARB) ± calcium-channel blockers form the main strategies for preventing its onset and slowing down its progression. Other strategies include uric acid antagonist, and renin and endothelin inhibitors. This book chapter discusses these predictive tools and possible preventive strategies.

Keywords: diabetic nephropathy, type 1 diabetes mellitus, type 2 diabetes mellitus, biomarkers, predictive tools, preventive strategies

1. Introduction

Type 1 diabetes mellitus is the usual form of diabetes mellitus in children. However, type 2 diabetes mellitus is now observed among them as well, especially in adolescents: with obesity as a putative risk factor. Diabetic nephropathy is the commonest microvascular complication of the kidney in both types of diabetes mellitus [1]. It is a clinical syndrome characterized by persistent macroalbuminuria (or urine albumin excretion rate of ≥200 μg/min) recorded at least twice within a 3- to 6-month interval, progressive decline in glomerular filtration rate (GFR), and hypertension [2]. The presence of microalbuminuria (urine albumin excretion rate of ≤199 μg/min) in type 1 diabetes mellitus is not only strongly predictive of macroalbuminuria (overt diabetic nephropathy) and subsequent end-stage renal disease (ESRD) but also constitutes a risk factor for future cardiovascular disease [3]. Contrary to the previously-held view that diabetic nephropathy is rare in childhood [4], some reports indicate that the disease can actually occur in the pediatric age group [5–7]. While the development of diabetic nephropathy can occur over a period of 10–20 years, beginning with microalbuminuria and ending with ESRD [1], it is currently projected that the rate of progression from microalbuminuria to macroalbuminuria over a 5- to 10-year period is about 15–30%, and may increase to 45% in patients with up to 15 years of diabetes duration [8].

Although microalbuminuria has traditionally remained the gold-standard biomarker for predicting diabetic nephropathy, its draw-backs include the following. Firstly, not all microalbuminuric diabetics will end up with diabetic nephropathy and ESRD [9, 10]. Secondly, microalbuminuria can only occur in the presence of significant renal injury since it is preceded by the appearance of several tubular and glomerular biomarkers in urine [11]. Thirdly, many diabetic patients with diabetic nephropathy can revert to normoalbuminuria, and these patients can also present with a reduction in GFR without progressing from normo- to macroalbuminuria (the concept of 'non-albuminuric' diabetic nephropathy) [12]. Thus, in place of microalbuminuria, these novel biomarkers are now increasingly used as earlier predictors of the disease.

In this book chapter, the use of biomarkers as predictive tools of diabetic nephropathy, and the preventive strategies against its onset and progression to ESRD are discussed.

1.1. Pathogenesis of diabetic nephropathy: a synopsis

In response to hyperglycemia, which disrupts the body's metabolic milieu, a cascade of complex molecular events occur resulting in the key pathogenic components of diabetic nephropathy, namely glomerular hypertrophy, tubular inflammation, mesangial expansion, oxidative stress, and renal fibrosis; several activated pathways individually or collectively influence the onset and progression of this disease [13]. However, it is important to note that genetic predisposition also contributes to the development of diabetic nephropathy because only 30–40% of diabetic patients develop diabetic kidney disease irrespective of glycemic control [14, 15].

In fact, the pathogenesis of the disease is based on a multifactorial interaction between metabolic and hemodynamic factors [16]. Metabolic factors involve glucose-dependent pathways, such as advanced glycation end-products and their receptors while hemodynamic factors consist of several vasoactive hormones, such as components of the renin–angiotensin system [16]. It is postulated that these metabolic and hemodynamic factors interact through common molecular and signaling pathways, such as protein kinase C leading to generation of reactive oxygen species. Presumably, these contributing factors result in pathological damage not only to the glomerulus, especially the podocytes, but also to the tubulo-interstitium. In other words, hyperglycemia induces vascular injury through complex overlapping pathways, comprising formation of advanced glycation end-products, activation of protein kinase C and generation of reactive oxygen species, which might play a key role in the initiation and progression of diabetic nephropathy [17].

Specifically, resident and nonresident cells of the kidney are stimulated by hyperglycemia to produce humoral mediators, cytokines, and growth factors which are implicated in the structural alterations such as increased deposition of extracellular matrix protein at the glomerulus, and functional alterations such as hyperpermeability of the glomerular basement membrane or shear stress [15]. Increased deposition of extracellular matrix protein results in basement membrane thickening and mesangial expansion while glomerular hyperpermeability leads to progressive albuminuria, which is one of the hallmarks of the disease (**Figure 1**).

1.2. Novel biomarkers as predictive tools for diabetic nephropathy

Novel biomarkers are now useful tools for predicting the onset and progression of diabetic nephropathy. Attempts have been made at classifying these biomarkers into major groups, although these groups overlap with one another. Representative groups include glomerular biomarkers; tubular biomarkers; biomarkers of inflammation; biomarkers of oxidative stress; and miscellaneous biomarkers [18]. Examples of each group of biomarkers include albumin, transferrin, laminin, immunoglobulin G, fibronectin, ceruloplasmin, type IV collagen, lipocalin-type prostaglandin synthase (L-PGDS), and glycosaminoglycans which make up the glomerular biomarkers; neutrophil gelatinase-associated lipocalin (NGAL), cystatin C, kidney molecule injury 1 (KIM-1), liver-type fatty acid binding protein (L-FABP),

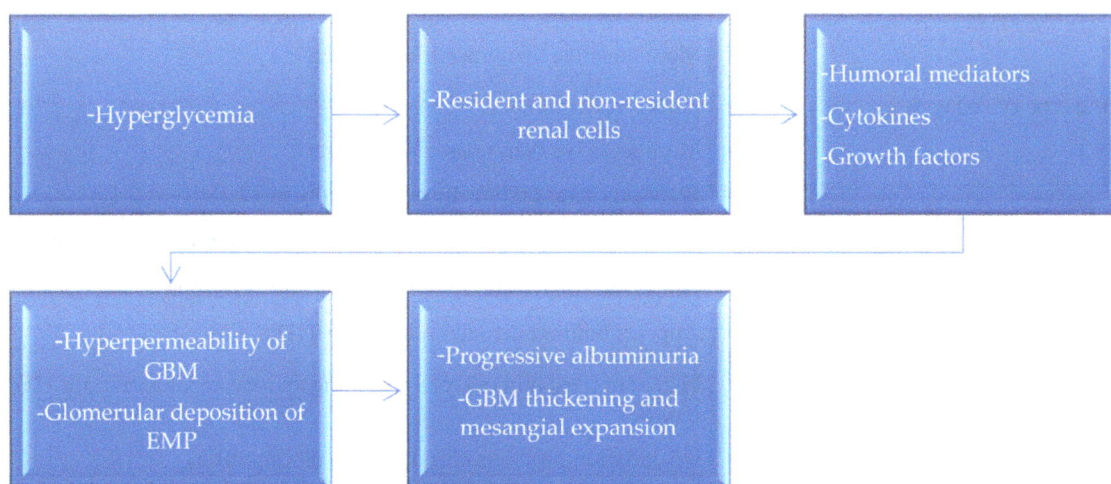

Figure 1. Pathogenetic pathway of albuminuria in diabetic nephropathy. GBM= glomerular basement membrane, EMP= extracellular matrix protein.

N-acetyl-β-D-glucosaminidase (NAG) and α-1-microglobulin constitute the tubular biomarkers; tumor necrosis factor-α (TNF-α), interleukin-1β, interleukin-8, interleukin-18, monocyte chemoattractant protein-1 (MCP-1), eotaxin, orosomucoid, RANTES and granulocyte colony-stimulating factor (G-CSF) represent the biomarkers of inflammation; 8-oxo-7,8-dihydro-2-deoxyguanosine (8oHdG) is a typical example of a biomarker of oxidative stress; nephrin, podocalyxin, advanced glycation end products (AGEs), vascular endothelial growth factor (VEGF), heart fatty-acid binding protein (H-FABP) and retinol-binding protein are listed as miscellaneous biomarkers. However, the overlap of the groups with one another shows that some miscellaneous biomarkers such as podocalyxin, nephrin and VEGF are also considered as glomerular biomarkers, whereas H-FABP and retinol-binding protein can be regarded as tubular biomarkers as well. Similarly, some biomarkers of inflammation such as TNF-α, the interleukins and MCP-1 are also identified as tubular biomarkers.

1.2.1. Glomerular biomarkers versus albuminuria

Several studies have provided evidence which indicate that novel glomerular biomarkers are more sensitive predictors of diabetic nephropathy compared to albuminuria, which has been considered as the conventional biomarker of glomerular injury (**Table 1**).

Firstly, urine transferrin, which is highly sensitive as a biomarker of diabetic nephropathy [19, 20], conversely has poor specificity for the disease because of confounders like primary

Glomerular biomarkers	Predictive ability for diabetic nephropathy
• Microalbuminuria	• Traditional biomarker predicting glomerular injury in T1DM and T2DM
• Urine transferrin	• High sensitivity
	• Poor specificity
	• More sensitive than microalbuminuria in predicting diabetic nephropathy in T2DM
• Urine ceruloplasmin	• High sensitivity
	• More sensitive than microalbuminuria
• Urine type IV collagen	• High sensitivity
	• More sensitive than microalbuminuria
	• Early predictor of diabetic nephropathy in T2DM
	• Can differentiate diabetic nephropathy from non-diabetic nephropathy
• Urine laminin	• Similar predictive ability with urine type IV collagen
	• Appears before microalbuminuria in T1DM
• Urine fibronectin	• Higher excretion in microalbuminuric than normoalbuminuric T2DM patients
	• Degradation products correlate with albuminuria

T1DM = type 1 diabetes mellitus, T2DM = type 2 diabetes mellitus.

Table 1. Glomerular biomarkers versus microalbuminuria as predictive tools for diabetic nephropathy.

glomerulonephritis and systemic diseases affecting the glomerulus, which also present with transferrinuria [21]. However, the biomarker is considered more sensitive than albuminuria. For instance, some authors have reported that, in the pre-albuminuric phase, transferrinuria was higher in diabetic subjects than in healthy controls [22, 23]. These findings underscore the superiority of urine transferrin over urine albumin excretion in the early prediction of diabetic nephropathy.

Secondly, urine ceruloplasmin is poorly filtered through the glomerular barrier because of its negative charge. Similar to urine transferrin, this biomarker can predict diabetic nephropathy earlier than albuminuria in patients with type 2 diabetes mellitus [24]. It has also been noted that urine ceruloplasmin together with urine transferrin, immunoglobulin G and orosomucoid are simultaneously elevated prior to the onset of microalbuminuria in type 2 diabetic patients [25].

Another remarkable glomerular biomarker is type IV collagen: a component of the glomerular basement membrane and mesangial matrix. Urine type IV collagen has been reported as a more sensitive marker of renal injury than urine albumin in patients with type 2 diabetes mellitus [26]. It can therefore serve an early predictor of diabetic nephropathy. Furthermore, urine type IV collagen can potentially differentiate diabetic nephropathy from non-diabetic nephropathy because studies show that type 2 diabetics with nephropathy have a significantly higher type IV collagen/albumin ratio in comparison with their non-diabetic cohorts with nephropathy [27, 28].

Laminin, a component of the glomerular basement membrane, is a biomarker with similar predictive properties as type IV collagen [29]. For instance, urine laminin can also discriminate between diabetic and non-diabetic nephropathy as one report showed that type 2 diabetics with nephropathy had significantly higher laminin/albumin ratio in comparison to patients with non-diabetic nephropathy [27]. More importantly, some investigators have documented a higher urine laminin excretion in pediatric patients with type 1 diabetes mellitus when juxtaposed with their healthy controls, even before the appearance of microalbuminuria [30].

Another glomerular biomarker worthy of mention is fibronectin. It is basically an intrinsic component of the glomerular extracellular matrix. Interestingly, urine fibronectin is reportedly higher in diabetic patients compared to their controls, with a significant difference noted only in macroalbuminuric patients [31, 32]. Further evidence supporting the predictive role of urine fibronectin in diabetic nephropathy include its higher excretion in type 2 diabetics with microalbuminuria than in those with normoalbuminuria [33], as well as the correlation of its degradation products with albuminuria [34].

1.2.2. Tubular biomarkers versus albuminuria

When compared to microalbuminuria and other novel glomerular biomarkers, tubular biomarkers are early predictors of diabetic nephropathy because tubulointerstitial lesions are known to occur much earlier in the course of the disease and may actually precede glomerular injury [35]. This characteristic has given this group of biomarkers an edge over glomerular biomarkers as earlier predictors of diabetic nephropathy.

For instance, studies on NGAL as a biomarker have revealed these interesting findings: presence of its elevated urine levels in diabetic patients with normoalbuminuria and its use in evaluating tubular lesions in the disease [36], its occurrence before microalbuminuria in patients with type 1 diabetes mellitus [37, 38], as well as its role in predicting the progression of diabetic kidney disease in type 2 diabetics [39, 40]. Thus, NGAL may have a better predictive ability for diabetic nephropathy than microalbuminuria.

Secondly, α-1-microglobulin has been identified as an affordable tubular biomarker for the early prediction of diabetic nephropathy [41]. Although α-1-microglobulin undergoes glomerular filtration, its tendency for proximal tubular reabsorption ensures its increased urine excretion in tubular dysfunction because of impaired reabsorption. In type 2 diabetics with normoalbuminuria, some authors were able to demonstrate increased urine levels of this biomarker because, as previously mentioned, tubular injury precedes the onset of microalbuminuria in diabetic nephropathy [42].

On the other hand, there appears to be divergent findings on the usefulness of NAG as a biomarker in the evaluation of diabetic nephropathy. Whereas some authors reported its clinical insignificance as an early biomarker of the disease [43], other reports conversely show that it remains a sensitive tubular biomarker for early detection of renal lesions in patients with both type 1 and 2 diabetes mellitus, as its urinary excretion can occur before microalbuminuria [44–46].

Furthermore, increased urine L-FABP levels have been observed in type 1 diabetics with normoalbuminuria, and is capable of not only predicting the onset of microalbuminuria but also its progression to macroalbuminuria [47]. Type 2 diabetics with normoalbuminuria also present with increased urine levels of this biomarker, which underscores its predictive ability for the onset and progression of diabetic nephropathy [48, 49].

Finally, some authors have reported the predictive ability of cystatin C for the progression of diabetic nephropathy [50], as well as its role in the evaluation of early nephropathy in type 2 diabetes mellitus [51], while increased urine KIM-1 levels have been observed more in diabetic patients with microalbuminuria than in those with normoalbuminuria [52]. This again suggests that tubular injury occurs early in the pathophysiologic trajectory of diabetic nephropathy.

1.2.3. Biomarkers of inflammation

Interestingly, the role of TNF-α (a pro-inflammatory cytokine) in the development of diabetic nephropathy is well documented [53–55]. The predictive ability of this cytokine as a biomarker for the disease is predicated upon the observations of its increased urine levels in diabetic patients who have albuminuria, as well as the significant rise of its urinary excretion during progression of diabetic nephropathy [54]. In fact, elevated urine TNF-α excretion and TNF-α levels in renal interstitial fluid have been noted to precede a significantly raised albuminuria in experimental diabetic rats [56]. This is corroborated by other studies which report a direct association between albuminuria and serum TNF-α in diabetic patients with normal renal function and microalbuminuria on one hand, as well as in those with macroalbuminuria and ESRD on the other hand [57, 58]. Similarly, other biomarkers of inflammation such as IL-8, MCP-1, G-CSF, eotaxin, and RANTES are reportedly higher in microalbuminuric type 2 diabetics than in their normoalbuminuric counterparts [59]. In type 1 diabetes mellitus, urine orosomucoid was also noted to be raised in normoalbuminuric patients when compared to non-diabetic controls: with increasing levels reported in microalbuminuric and macroalbuminuric diabetic patients [60].

1.2.4. Biomarkers of oxidative stress

8oHdG is the prototype of this group of biomarkers. This molecule is actually a product of oxidative injury to DNA which appears unchanged in the urine. It may represent a dependable clinical biomarker for predicting the onset of diabetic kidney disease because some authors have observed that patients whose nephropathy progressed significantly had higher urinary excretion of this biomarker than those who had lower or moderate urinary excretion [61].

2. Preventive strategies for diabetic nephropathy

Generally, strict glycemic control and painstaking control of hypertension have significant impact on prevention and progression of diabetic nephropathy; a finding noted in adult patients with type 2 diabetes mellitus [62]. In children and adolescents, who are predominantly type 1 diabetics, these measures should be equally applicable as preventive strategies. More importantly, strategies that target the modifiable risk factors for diabetic nephropathy may result in better outcomes. Some of the modifiable and non-modifiable risk factors include poor glycemic control, pubertal growth spurt, hypertension, hyperlipidemia, smoking habits, albuminuria, obesity and genetic predisposition [6, 63–66]. For instance, in type 1 diabetes mellitus, strict glycemic control is the major preventive strategy for diabetic nephropathy, whereas in type 2 diabetes mellitus, modulation of hypertension, dyslipidemia, and obesity (modifiable risk factors) constitute important strategies [63]. Notably, the current recommendations/strategies for preventing the onset and retarding the progression of diabetic nephropathy are essentially evidence-based, and are summarized in **Table 2**.

Firstly, the measurement of hemoglobin A1 c (Hb A1 c) has been adopted as a reliable tool for assessing glycemic control. It is a marker for average glycemic levels over the previous 3 months. The goal of glycemic control is basically to maintain Hb A1 c level of less than 7% while avoiding hypoglycemia. In fact, strict glycemic control reduces the risk of microvascular complications in both type 1 and type 2 diabetes mellitus [67, 68]. Reports show that diabetic nephropathy rarely occurs when the Hb A1 c level is consistently less than 7.5–8.0% [2, 65]. Notably, results of two major clinical trials have buttressed the effectiveness of tight glycemic control as a preventive strategy [68, 69]. In one of the studies conducted on type 2 diabetics, there was a 34% reduction in the risk of microalbuminuria [68], while in type 1 diabetics, the incidence of microalbuminuria was decreased by 39% in the primary prevention group with a 54% reduction in its progression to macroalbuminuria in the secondary prevention group [69].

Secondly, the control of hypertension is renoprotective in type 1 and type 2 diabetes mellitus, as it reduces albuminuria and delays the onset of nephropathy [70]. The renin-angiotensin system constitutes the target of the most effective strategy for blood-pressure control and for reducing the pathophysiologic abnormalities which lead to albuminuria. Specifically, it

Preventive strategies	Mechanism of action
• Strict or tight glycemic control	• Reduces risk of microalbuminuria
	• Reduces progression of microalbuminuria to macroalbuminuria
• Antihypertensive therapy with ACEI/ARB ± calcium-channel blockers	• Reduces albuminuria and delays the onset of diabetic nephropathy
	• Prevents progression of diabetic nephropathy in microalbuminuric patients
• Vitamin D	• Ameliorates nephropathy by reducing albuminuria
• Allopurinol (uric acid antagonist)	• Reduces urinary TGF-β in diabetic nephropathy
• Aliskiren (renin inhibitor)	• Reduces albuminuria and serves as an antihypertensive in T2DM
• Atrasentan (endothelial inhibitor)	• Reduces residual albuminuria in type 2 diabetic nephropathy
• Dietary protein/phosphate restriction	• Retards progression of diabetic nephropathy

ACEI = angiotensin-converting enzyme inhibitor, ARB = angiotensin-receptor blocker, TGF-β = transforming growth factor-beta, T2DM = type 2 diabetes mellitus.

Table 2. Preventive strategies for the onset and progression of diabetic nephropathy: an evidence-based summary.

does appear that blood pressure elevation directly correlates with the degree of albuminuria in type 2 diabetes mellitus [71]. Thus, antihypertensive therapy, especially with angiotensin converting enzyme inhibitors (ACEI) or in combination with other antihypertensive agents, is an effective strategy for preventing the progression of diabetic nephropathy [71]. While either ACEI or angiotensin-II type 1 receptor blockers (ARB) is recommended in patients with microalbuminuria and type 2 diabetes mellitus [72], none of them is recommended in normotensive, normoalbuminuric diabetics for the primary prevention of diabetic nephropathy. Apart from ACEI which are regarded as first-choice treatment for hypertension in diabetics, other effective alternative antihypertensive drugs include calcium-channel blockers: either alone [73], or in combination with ACEI [74].

Thirdly, the use of novel treatments has been tried as strategies for preventing the onset and progression of diabetic nephropathy. These therapeutic agents include the following: vitamin D, allopurinol (uric acid antagonist), aliskiren (renin inhibitor), and atrasentan (endothelin antagonist or l inhibitor) [75–78]. In experimental murine models, vitamin D is thought to activate an antioxidant pathway and ameliorate diabetic nephropathy by reducing albuminuria [75]. Furthermore, vitamin D deficiency is known to be a common disorder in diabetics and probably constitutes a risk factor for ischemic heart disease, worsening of chronic kidney disease and diabetic nephropathy [79]. Vitamin D metabolites may inhibit the renin-angiotensin system and exert renoprotective effect by preventing glomerulosclerosis and reducing albuminuria in diabetic nephropathy; in addition, administering the vitamin is reported to have resulted in a reduction in insulin resistance and blood pressure [80, 81]. In fact, findings from several studies support the beneficial effect of dietary or supplemental vitamin D in retarding the progression of diabetic nephropathy through reduction of albuminuria [82–85]. Another novel therapeutic agent- allopurinol- was reported to reduce albuminuria in patients with type 2 diabetes [86]. Evidence point to a greater serum uric acid level in patients with diabetic nephropathy than in normal subjects [87]. Uric acid specifically plays a mediatory role in the pathogenesis of diabetic nephropathy, as it leads to endothelial dysfunction, increased activity of the renin-angiotensin-aldosterone system (RAAS), and induction of inflammatory cascades, as well as profibrotic cytokine activation which synergistically contribute to progression of microvascular disease and extracellular matrix deposition; these events result in kidney injury in diabetic nephropathy [87]. Obviously, hyperuricemia may thus impair glomerular function, and promote albuminuria. Interestingly, allopurinol has also been observed to reduce urinary transforming growth factor-beta (TGF-β) in diabetic nephropathy, apart from improving endothelial dysfunction [76]. Furthermore, the direct renin inhibitor-aliskiren-reportedly reduces albuminuria and also serves as an antihypertensive in type 2 diabetes mellitus either as a monotherapy [77], or in combination with an angiotensin receptor blocker (ARB) [88]. Endothelin-1 is regarded as the most potent vasoconstrictor which plays a role in renal regulation of fluid and salt balance. More importantly, excessive renal production of endothelin-1 is associated with proteinuria and tubulointerstitial injury [89]. Although trials are still going on to validate the endothelin antagonist or inhibitor (atrasentan), this novel agent has been shown to lower residual albuminuria in type 2 diabetic nephropathy besides its antihypertensive action [78].

Finally, dietary modification has proved to be an effective tool in retarding the progression of diabetic nephropathy. In diabetics, high dietary protein has renal hemodynamic effects which comprise elevated GFR, hyperfiltration, and raised intraglomerular pressure which are probably accentuated by poor glycemic control [79]. Thus, it has been observed that dietary protein restriction slows down the deterioration of kidney function in type 1 and type 2 diabetes mellitus [90, 91]. For instance, a prospective study which compared type 1 diabetics placed on dietary protein/phosphate restriction with those on unrestricted diet revealed a differential reduction in GFR, as the GFR in the former group was progressively reduced by only 0.26 ml/min/month compared with 1.01 ml/min/month seen in the latter group [92].

3. Conclusion

Both glomerular and tubular biomarkers are sensitive predictors of diabetic nephropathy when compared to microalbuminuria, with tubular biomarkers serving as earlier predictors of the disease. Other groups of novel biomarkers have also been shown to be effective predictive tools. As the major microvascular complication of both type 1 and type 2 diabetes mellitus and an important cause of ESRD-related mortality, the onset and progression of diabetic nephropathy therefore constitute an important challenge in diabetic care. Fortunately, strict glycemic control and antihypertensive therapy with ACEI/ARB ± calcium-channel blockers form the main strategies for preventing the onset and slowing the progression of diabetic nephropathy. Other novel treatment options include dietary protein restriction, use of vitamin D, uric acid antagonist, as well as renin and endothelin inhibitors. As newer strategies emerge, prospects for better outcomes in diabetic nephropathy are getting brighter.

Acknowledgements

The authors acknowledge the useful information obtained from the cited paper- SN Uwaezuoke (2015) Prevention of Diabetic Nephropathy in Children and Adolescents: How Effective are the Current Strategies? Int J Diabetol Vasc Dis Res, S5:001, 1-5.

Conflict of interest

The authors declare no conflict of interests in this work.

Author details

Samuel N. Uwaezuoke[1,2]*, Ugo N. Chikani[1,2] and Ngozi R. Mbanefo[2]

*Address all correspondence to: samuel.uwaezuoke@unn.edu.ng

1 College of Medicine, University of Nigeria/University of Nigeria Teaching Hospital, Enugu, Ituku-Ozalla, Nigeria

2 University of Nigeria Teaching Hospital, Enugu, Ituku-Ozalla, Nigeria

References

[1] Koulouridis E. Diabetic nephropathy in children and adolescents and its consequences in adults. Journal of Pediatric Endocrinology and Metabolism. 2001;**14**:S1367-S1377. PMID: 11964036

[2] Deferrari G, Repetto M, Calvi C, Ciabattoni M, Rossi C, Robaudo C. Diabetic nephropathy: From micro- to microalbuminuria. Nephrology, Dialysis and Transplantation. 1998;**13**:S11-S15. PMID: 9870419

[3] McKenna K, Thompson C. Microalbuminuria: A marker to increased renal and cardiovascular risk in diabetes mellitus. Scottish Medical Journal. 1997;**42**:99-104

[4] Danne T, Kordonouri O, Hövener G, Weber B. Diabetic angiopathy in children. Dia betic Medicine. 1997;**14**:1012-1025. DOI: 10.1002/(SICI)1096-9136(199712)14:12<1012:AID-DIA479>3.0.CO;2-H

[5] DeClue TJ, Campos A. Diabetic nephropathy in a prepubertal diabetic female. Journal of Pediatric Endocrinology. 1994;**7**:43-46. PMID: 8186823

[6] Maghribi H, Abu-Odeh A. Early diabetic nephropathy in a pediatric patient. Journal of the Royal Medical Services. 2006;**13**:51-53

[7] Francis J, Rose SJ, Raafat F, Milford DV. Early onset of diabetic nephropathy. Archives of diseases in childhood. 1997;**77**:524-525. PMCID: PMC1717409

[8] Caramori ML, Fioretto P, Mauer M. Enhancing the predictive value of urinary albumin for diabetic nephropathy. Journal of the American Society of Nephrology. 2006;**17**:339-352. DOI: 10.1681/ASN.2005101075

[9] Remuzzi G, Schieppati A, Ruggenenti P. Nephropathy in patients with type 2 diabetes. New England Journal of Medicine. 2002;**346**:1145-1115. DOI: 10.1056/NEJMcp011773

[10] Adler AI, Stevens RJ, Manley SE, Bilous RW, Cull CA, Holman RR; UKPDS GROUP. Development and progression of nephropathy in type 2 diabetes: The United Kingdom prospective diabetes study (UKPDS 64). Kidney International. 2003;**63**:225-232. DOI: 10.1046/j.1523-1755.2003.00712.x

[11] Matheson A, Willcox MDP, Flanagan J, Walsh BJ. Urinary biomarkers involved in type 2 diabetes: A review. Diabetes Metabolism Research and Reviews. 2010;**26**:150-171. DOI: 10.1002/dmrr.1068

[12] Currie G, McKay G, Delles C. Biomarkers in diabetic nephropathy: Present and future. World Journal of Diabetes. 2014;**5**:763-776. DOI: 10.4239/wjd.v5.i6.763

[13] Arora MK, Singh UK. Molecular mechanisms in the pathogenesis of diabetic nephropathy: An update. Vascular Pharmacology. 2013;**58**:259-271. DOI: 10.1016/j.vph.2013.01.001

[14] The Diabetes Control and Complications (DCCT) Research Group: Effect of intensive therapy on the development and progression of diabetic nephropathy in the diabetes control and complications trial. Kidney International. 1995;**47**:1703-1720. PMID: 7643540

[15] Schena FP, Gesualdo L. Pathogenetic mechanisms of diabetic nephropathy. Journal of American Society Nephrology. 2005;**16**:S30-S33. PMID: 15938030

[16] Cao Z, Cooper ME. Pathogenesis of diabetic nephropathy. Journal of Diabetes Investi gation. 2011;**2**:243-247. DOI: 10.1111/j.2040-1124.2011.00131.x

[17] Forbes JM, Coughlan MT, Cooper ME. Oxidative stress as a major culprit in kidney disease in diabetes. Diabetes. 2008;**57**:1446-1454. DOI: 10.2337/db08-0057

[18] Uwaezuoke SN. The role of novel biomarkers in predicting diabetic nephropathy: A review. International Journal of Nephrology and Renovascular Disease. 2017;**10**:221-231. DOI: 10.2147/IJNRD.S143186

[19] Bernard AM, Amor AA, Goemaere-Vanneste J, et al. Microtransferrinuria is a more sensitive indicator of early glomerular damage in diabetes than microalbuminuria. Clinical Chemistry. 1988;**34**:1920-1921. PMID: 3416456

[20] O'Donnell MJ, Martin P, Cavan D, et al. Increased urinary transferrin excretion in exercising normoalbuminuric insulin-dependent diabetic patients. Annals of Clinical Biochemistry. 1991;**28**:456-460. DOI: 10.1177/000456329102800506

[21] Yaqoob M, McClelland P, Patrick AW, Stevenson A, Mason H, Bell GM. Tubular damage in microalbuminuric patients with primary glomerulonephritis and diabetic nephropathy. Renal Failure. 1995;**17**:43-49. PMID: 7770643

[22] Martin P, Walton C, Chapman C, Bodansky HJ, Stickland MH. Increased urinary excretion of transferrin in children with type 1 diabetes mellitus. Diabetic Medicine. 1990;**7**: 35-40. PMID: 1688749

[23] Cheung CK, Cockram CS, Yeung VT, Swaminathan R. Urinary excretion of transferrin by non-insulin-dependent diabetics: A marker for early complications? Clinical Chemistry. 1989;**35**:1672-1674. PMID: 2758634

[24] Wang C, Li C, Gong W, Lou T. New urinary biomarkers for diabetic kidney disease. Biomarker Research. 2013;**1**:9. DOI: 10.1186/2050-7771-1-9

[25] Narita T, Sasaki H, Hosoba M, et al. Parallel increase in urinary excretion rates of immunoglobulin G, ceruloplasmin, transferrin, and orosomucoid in normoalbuminuric type 2 diabetic patients. Diabetes Care. 2004;**27**:1176-1181. PMID: 15111541

[26] Kotajima N, Kimura T, Kanda T, et al. Type IV collagen as an early marker for diabetic nephropathy in non- insulin-dependent diabetes mellitus. The Journal of Diabetic Complications. 2000;**14**:13-17. PMID: 10925061

[27] Banu N, Hara H, Okamura M, Egusa G, Yamakido M. Urinary excretion of type IV collagen and laminin in the evaluation of nephropathy in NIDDM: Comparison with urinary albumin and markers of tubular dysfunction and/or damage. Diabetes Research and Clinical Practice. 1995;**29**:57-67. DOI: 10.1016/0168-8227(95)01119-X

[28] Kado S, Aoki A, Wada S, et al. Urinary type IV collagen as a marker for early diabetic nephropathy. Diabetes Research and Clinical Practice. 1996;**31**:103-108. DOI: 10.1016/0168-8227(96)01210-7

[29] Haiyashi Y, Makino H, Ota Z. Serum and urinary concentrations of type IV collagen and laminin as a marker of microangiopathy in diabetes. Diabetic Medicine. 1992;**9**:366-370. PMID: 1600709

[30] Miyake H, Nagashima K, Yagi H, Onigata K. Urinary laminin P1 as an index of glycemic control in children with insulin-dependent diabetes mellitus. Diabetes Research. 1992;**23**:131-138. PMID: 7536137

[31] Fagerudd JA, Groop PH, Honkanen E, Teppo AM, Grönhagen-Riska C. Urinary excretion of TGF-β1, PDGF-BB and fibronectin in insulin-dependent diabetes mellitus patients. Kidney International. 1997;**51**:S195-S197

[32] Kanauchi M, Nishioka H, Hashimoto T, Dohi K. Diagnostic significance of urinary transferrin in diabetic nephropathy. Nihon Jinzo Gakkai Shi. 1995;**37**:649-654. PMID: 8583702

[33] Takahashi M. Increased urinary fibronectin excretion in type II diabetic patients with microalbuminuria. Nihon Jinzo Gakkai Shi. 1995;**37**:336-342. PMID: 8583702

[34] Kuboki K, Tada H, Shin K, Oshima Y, Isogai S. Relationship between urinary excretion of fibronectin degradation products and proteinuria in diabetic patients, and their

suppression after continuous subcutaneous heparin infusion. Diabetes Research and Clinical Practice. 1993;**21**:61-66. PMID: 8253024

[35] Mise K, Hoshino J, Ueno T, et al. Prognostic value of tubulointerstitial lesions, urinary N-acetylβ-d-glucosaminidase, and urinary β2-microglobulin in patients with type 2 diabetes and biopsy-proven diabetic nephropathy. Clinical Journal of the American Society of Nephrology. 2016;**11**:593-601. DOI: 10.2215/CJN.04980515

[36] Lacquaniti A, Donato V, Pintaudi B, et al. "Normoalbuminuric" diabetic nephropathy: Tubular damage and NGAL. Acta Diabetologica. 2013;**50**:935-942. DOI: 10.1007/s00592-013-0485-7

[37] Bolignano D, Lacquaniti A, Coppolino G, et al. Neutrophil gelatinase-associated lipocalin as an early biomarker of nephropathy in diabetic patients. Kidney and Blood Pressure Research. 2009;**32**:91-98. DOI: 10.1159/000209379

[38] Yürük Yıldırım Z, Nayır A, Yılmaz A, Gedikbası A, Bundak R. Neutrophil gelatinase-associated lipocalin as an early sign of diabetic kidney injury in children. Journal of Clinical Research and Pediatric Endocrinology. 2015;**7**:274-279. DOI: 10.4274/jcrpe.2002

[39] Yang YH, He XJ, Chen SR, Wang L, Li EM, Xu LY. Changes of serum and urine neutrophil gelatinase-associated lipocalin in type-2 diabetic patients with nephropathy: One year observational follow-up study. Endocrine. 2009;**36**:45-51. DOI: 10.1007/s12020-009-9187-x

[40] de Carvalho JA, Tatsch E, Hausen BS, et al. Urinary kidney injury molecule-1 and neutrophil gelatinase-associated lipocalin as indicators of tubular damage in normoalbuminuric patients with type 2 diabetes. Clinical Biochemistry. 2016;**49**:232-236. DOI: 10.1016/j.clinbiochem.2015.10.016

[41] Shore N, Khurshid R, Saleem M. Alpha-1-microglobulin: A marker for early detection of tubular disorders in diabetic nephropathy. Journal of Ayub Medical College Abbottabad. 2010;**22**:53-55

[42] Hong CY, Hughes K, Chia KS, Ng V, Ling SL. Urinary alpha-1-microglobulin as a marker of nephropathy in type 2 diabetic Asian subjects in Singapore. Diabetes Care. 2003;**26**:338-342. PMID: 12547859

[43] Ambade V, Singh P, Somani BL, Basannar D. Urinary N-acetyl β-glucosaminidase and γ-glutamyl transferase as early markers of diabetic nephropathy. Indian Journal of Clinical Biochemistry. 2006;**2**:142-148. DOI: 10.1007/BF02912930

[44] Patel DN, Kalia K. Efficacy of urinary N-acetyl-β-D glucosaminidase to evaluate early renal tubular damage as a consequence of type 2 diabetes mellitus: A cross-sectional study. International Journal of Diabetes in Developing Countries. 2015;**35**:449-457. DOI: 10.1007/s13410-015-0404-2

[45] Assal HS, Tawfeek S, Rasheld EA, El-Lebedy D, Thabet EH. Serum cystatin C and tubular urinary enzymes as biomarkers: A renal dysfunction in type 2 diabetes mellitus. Clinical Medicine Insights: Endocrinology and Diabetes. 2013;**6**:7-13. DOI: 10.4137/CMED.S12633

[46] Jones AP, Lock S, Griffiths KD. Urinary N-acetyl-β-glucosaminidase activity in type I diabetes mellitus. Annals of Clinical Biochemistry. 1995;**32**:58-62. DOI: 10.1177/000456 329503200104

[47] Nielsen SE, Sugaya T, Hovind P, et al. Urinary liver-type fatty acid-binding protein predicts progression to nephropathy in type 1 diabetic patients. Diabetes Care. 2010;**33**:1320-1324. DOI: 10.2337/dc09-2242

[48] Kamijo-Ikemori A, Sugaya T, Yasuda T, et al. Clinical significance of urinary liver-type fatty acid-binding protein in diabetic nephropathy of type 2 diabetic patients. Diabetes Care. 2011;**34**:691-696. DOI: 10.2337/dc10-1392

[49] Panduru NM, Forsblom C, Saraheimo M, et al., Finn Diane Study Group. Urinary liver-type fatty acid binding protein and progression of diabetic nephropathy in type 1 diabetes. Diabetes Care. 2013;**36**:2077-2083. DOI: 10.2337/dc12-1868

[50] Kim SS, Song SH, Kim IJ, et al. Urinary cystatin C and tubular proteinuria predict progression of diabetic nephropathy. Diabetes Care. 2013;**36**:656-661. DOI: 10.2337/dc12-0849

[51] Jeon YK, Kim MR, Huh JE, et al. Cystatin C as an early biomarker of nephropathy in patients with type 2 diabetes. Journal of Korean Medical Sciences. 2011;**26**:258-263. DOI: 10.3346/jkms.2011.26.2.258

[52] Petrica L, Vlad A, Gluhovschi G, et al. Proximal tubule dysfunction is associated with podocyte damage biomarkers nephrin and vascular endothelial growth factor in type 2 diabetes mellitus patients: A cross-sectional study. PLoS One. 2014;**9**:e112538. DOI: 10.1371/journal.pone.0112538

[53] Elmarakby AA, Sullivan JC. Relationship between oxidative stress and inflammatory cytokines in diabetic nephropathy. Cardiovascular Therapeutics. 2012;**30**:49-59. DOI: 10.1111/j.1755-5922.2010.00218.x

[54] Navarro JF, Mora C. Diabetes, inflammation, proinflammatory cytokines, and diabetic nephropathy. The Scientific World Journal. 2006;**6**:908-917. DOI: 10.1100/tsw.2006.179

[55] Hasegawa G, Nakano K, Sawada M, et al. Possible role of tumor necrosis factor and interleukin-1 in the development of diabetic nephropathy. Kidney International. 1991;**40**:1007-1012. PMID: 1762301

[56] Kalantarinia K, Awas AS, Siragy HM. Urinary and renal interstitial concentrations of TNF-α increase prior to the rise in albuminuria in diabetic rats. Kidney International. 2003;**64**:1208-1213. DOI: 10.1046/j.1523-1755.2003.00237.x

[57] Navarro JF, Mora C, Maca M, Garca J. Inflammatory parameters are independently associated with urinary albumin excretion in type 2 diabetes mellitus. American Journal of Kidney Diseases. 2003;**42**:53-61. PMID: 12830456

[58] Navarro JF, Mora C, Rivero A, et al. Urinary protein excretion and serum tumor necrosis factor in diabetic patients with advanced renal failure: Effects of pentoxifylline administration. American Journal of Kidney Diseases. 1999;**33**:458-463

[59] Liu J, Zhao Z, Willcox MD, Xu B, Shi B. Multiplex bead analysis of urinary cytokines of type 2 diabetic patients with normo- and microalbuminuria. Journal of Immunoassay and Immunochemistry. 2010;31:279-289. DOI: 10.1080/15321819.2010.524860

[60] Jiang H, Guan G, Zhang R, et al. Increased urinary excretion of orosomucoid is a risk predictor of diabetic nephropathy. Nephrology. 2009;14:332-337. DOI: 10.1111/j.1440-1797.2008.01053.x

[61] Hinokio Y, Suzuki S, Hirai M, Suzuki C, Suzuki M, Toyota T. Urinary excretion of 8-oxo-7,8-dihydro-2-deoxyguanosine as a predictor of the development of diabetic nephropathy. Diabetologia. 2002;45:877-882. DOI: 10.1007/s00125-002-0831-8

[62] O'Connor PJ, Spann SJ, Woolf SH. Care of adults with type 2 diabetes mellitus: A review of the evidence. Journal of Family Practice. 1988;47:S13-S22. PMID: 9834750

[63] Molnár M, Wittmann I, Nagy J. Prevalence, course and risk factors of diabetic nephropathy in type-2 diabetes mellitus. Medical Science Monitor. 2000;6:929-936. PMID: 11208433

[64] Bogdanović R. Diabetic nephropathy in children. Nephrology, Dialysis and Transplantation.2001;16:S120-S122. PMID: 11568268

[65] Di Landro D, Catalano C, Lambertini D, et al. The effect of metabolic control on development and progression of diabetic nephropathy. Nephrology, Dialysis and Transplantation. 1988;13:S35-S43. PMID: 9870424

[66] Sochett E, Daneman D. Early diabetes-related complication in children and adolescents with type 1 diabetes. Implications for screening and intervention. Endocrinology and Metabolism Clinics of North America. 1999;28:865-882. PMID: 10609124

[67] Molitch ME. The relationship between glucose control and the development of diabetic nephropathy in type I diabetes. Seminars in Nephrology. 1997;17:101-113. PMID: 9148376

[68] UK Prospective Diabetes Study Group. Intensive blood-glucose control with sulphonylureas or insulin compared with conventional treatment and risk of complications in patients with type 2 diabetes (UKPDS 33). Lancet. 1998;352:837-853. PMID: 9742976

[69] The Diabetes Control and Complications Trial Research Group. The effect of intensive treatment of diabetes on the development and progression of long-term complications in insulin-dependent diabetes mellitus. New England Journal of Medicine. 1993;329:977-986. DOI: 10.1056/NEJM199309303291401

[70] Parving HH. Is antihypertensive treatment the same for NIDDM and IDDM patients? Diabetes Research and Clinical Practice. 1998;39:S43-S47. PMID: 9649959

[71] Mogensen CE. Drug treatment for hypertensive patients in special situations: Diabetes and hypertension. Clinical and Experimental Hypertension. 1999;21:895-906. PMID: 10423111

[72] Jerums G, MacIsaac RJ. Treatment of microalbuminuria in patients with type 2 diabetes mellitus. Treatment in Endocrinology. 2002;1:163-173. PMID: 15799209

[73] Rossing P. Promotion, prediction and prevention of progression of nephropathy in type 1 diabetes mellitus. Diabetic Medicine. 1998;15:900-919. DOI: 10.1002/(SICI)1096-9136(1998110)15:11<900::AID-DIA709>3.0.CO;2-0

[74] Bakris GL, Weir MR, DeQuattro V, McMahon FG. Effects of an ACE inhibitor/calcium antagonist combination on proteinuria in diabetic nephropathy. Kidney International. 1998;54:1283-1289. DOI: 10.1046/j.1523-1755.1998.00083.x

[75] Nakai K, Fujii H, Kono K, et al. Vitamin D activates the Nrf2-Keap1 antioxidant pathway and ameliorates nephropathy in diabetic rats. American Journal of Hypertension. 2014;27:586-595. DOI: 10.1093/ajh/hpt160

[76] Talaat KM. el-sheikh AR. The effect of mild hyperuricemia on urinary transforming growth factor beta and the progression of chronic kidney disease. American Journal of Nephrology. 2007;27:435-440. DOI: 10.1159/000105142

[77] Persson F, Rossing P, Schjoedt KJ, et al. Time course of the antiproteinuric and antihypertensive effects of direct renin inhibition in type 2 diabetes. Kidney International. 2008;73:1419-1425. DOI: 10.1038/ki.2008.68

[78] de Zeeuw D, Coll B, Andress D, et al. The endothelial antagonist atrasentan lowers residual albuminuria in patients with type 2 diabetic nephropathy. Journal of American Society of Nephrology. 2014;25:1083-1093. DOI: 10.1681/ASN.2013080830

[79] Diaz VA, Mainous AG 3rd, Carek PJ, Wessell AM, Everett CJ. The association of vitamin D deficiency and insufficiency with diabetic nephropathy: Implications for health disparities. Journal of American Board of Family Medicine. 2009;22:521-527

[80] Zhang Z, Sun L, Wang Y, et al. Renoprotective role of the vitamin D receptor in diabetic nephropathy. Kidney International. 2008;73:163-171. DOI: 10.1038/sj.ki.5002572

[81] Schwarz U, Amann K, Orth SR, Simonaviciene A, Wessels S, Ritz E. Effect of 1,25 (OH)2 vitamin D3 on glomerulosclerosis in subtotally nephrectomized rats. Kidney International. 1998;53:1696-1705. DOI: 10.1046/j.15231755.1998.00951.x

[82] Kim MJ, Frankel AH, Donaldson M, et al. Oral cholecalciferol decreases albuminuria and urinary TGF-beta1 in patients with type 2 diabetic nephropathy on established renin angiotensin-aldosterone system inhibition. Kidney International. 2011;80:851-860

[83] Bonakdaran S, Hami M, Hatefi A. The effects of calcitriol on albuminuria in patients with type-2 diabetes mellitus. Saudi Journal of Kidney Diseases and Transplantation. 2012;23:121520. DOI: 10.4103/1319-2442.103562

[84] de Zeeuw D, Agarwal R, Amdahl M, et al. Selective vitamin D receptor activation with paricalcitol for reduction of albuminuria in patients with type 2 diabetes (VITAL study): A randomized controlled trial. Lancet. 2010;376(9752):1543-1551. DOI: 10.1016/S01406736(10)61032-X

[85] Huang Y, Yu H, Lu J, et al. Oral supplementation with cholecalciferol 800 IU ameliorates albuminuria in Chinese type 2 diabetic patients with nephropathy. PLoS One. 2012;7(11):e50510. DOI: 10.1371/journal.pone.0050510

[86] Momeni A, Shahidi S, Seirafian S, Taheri S, Kheiri S. Effect of allopurinol in decreasing proteinuria in type 2 diabetic patients. Iranian Journal of Kidney Diseases. 2010;4:128-132

[87] Jalal DI, Maahs DM, Hovind P, Nakagawa T. Uric acid as a mediator of diabetic nephropathy. Seminars in Nephrology. 2011;31:459-465. DOI: 10.1016/j. semnephrol.2011.08.011

[88] Parving HH, Persson F, Lewis JB, Lewis EJ, Hollenberg NK. Aliskiren combined with losartan in type 2 diabetes and nephropathy. New England Journal of Medicine. 2008;358:243346. DOI: 10.1056/NEJMoa0708379

[89] Egido J, Rojas-Rivera J, Mas S, et al. Atrasentan for the treatment of diabetic nephropathy. Expert Opinion on Investigational Drugs. 2017;26:741-750. DOI: 10.1080/13543784. 2017.1325872

[90] Evans TC, Capell P. Diabetic nephropathy. Clinical Diabetes. 2000;18:1-16

[91] Barsotti G, Cupisti A, Barsotti M, et al. Dietary treatment of diabetic nephropathy with chronic renal failure. Nephrology, Dialysis and Transplantation. 1998;13:49-52. PMID: 9870426

[92] Toeller M, Buyken AE. Protein intake–new evidence for its role in diabetic nephropathy. Nephrology, Dialysis and Transplantation. 1998;13:1926-1927. PMID: 9719140

6

Towards Metabolic Biomarkers for the Diagnosis and Prognosis of CKD

Ulrika Lundin and Klaus M. Weinberger

Abstract

Chronic kidney disease, the gradual loss of renal function, is an increasingly recognized burden for patients and health care systems; globally, it has a high and rapidly growing prevalence, a significant mortality, and causes disproportionately high costs, particularly for hemodialysis and kidney transplantations. Yet, the available diagnostic tools are either impractical in clinical routine or have serious shortcomings preventing a well-informed disease management, although optimized treatment strategies with impressive benefits for patients have been established. Advances in bioanalytics have facilitated the identification of many genomic, proteomic, and metabolic biomarker candidates, some of which have been validated in independent cohorts. Summarizing the markers discovered so far, this chapter focuses on compounds or pathways, for which quantitative data, substantiating evidence from translational research, and a mechanistic understanding is available. Also, multiparametric marker panels have been suggested with promising diagnostic and prognostic performance in initial analyses, although the data basis from prospective trials is very limited. Large-scale studies, however, are underway and will validate certain sets of parameters and discard others. Finally, the path from clinical research to routine application is discussed, focusing on potential obstacles such as the use of mass spectrometry, and the feasibility of obtaining regulatory approval for metabolomics assays.

Keywords: metabolomics, biomarkers, diabetic nephropathy, diagnosis, prognosis

1. Introduction: innovation in laboratory diagnostics

Most technological innovations go through typical cycles of acceptance and spread, the so-called innovation curves, quite generically analyzed by Rogers [1]. The same is true for new bioanalytical techniques or methods, which typically trigger a phase of early adoption and rather untargeted exploration of their use in many different areas (basic and applied research, drug development, clinical diagnostics, etc.). Some of these new technologies were able to make significant inroads in routine diagnostics within years of their invention, for example, immunoassays [2] based on monoclonal antibodies [3], Southern and Western blotting [4, 5], the polymerase chain reaction [6], or nucleic acid sequencing by chain termination [7], while others have been well-developed and contributed to major scientific successes for decades without being adopted in clinical routine, for example, Raman, infrared, or nuclear magnetic resonance (NMR) spectroscopy (*nota bene*, the latter succeeded as a disruptive new imaging modality in radiology instead of clinical chemistry).

The discovery, development, and validation of new diagnostic markers and of assays for their standardized detection are a very costly endeavor that can only be successful after diligent analysis of all relevant boundary conditions (medical, ethical, technological, commercial, etc.). The first and foremost question in this analysis is, of course, if there is an unmet medical need for more and/or different information about a patient's status, for example, describing the actual pathophysiological alterations with greater diagnostic accuracy, predicting the course of the disease or the response to certain treatments earlier or with improved predictive values, or keeping track of the beneficial or harmful effects of any therapeutic interventions (clinical, pharmacodynamic, or pharmacokinetic monitoring [8]).

In this context, it should go without saying that additional diagnostic data points are only clinically valuable—and justify product development by companies and reimbursement by public health care systems—if there is a rather immediate therapeutic consequence, that is, if treatment or disease management are guided in a way that would not be possible without this information. Producing diagnostic data without a clinical consequence must be seen as a dubious way of stretching the already tight budgets of health care systems and insurances, and may even be problematic in terms of medical ethics, for example, in newborn screening for metabolic disorders, where signatures indicative of many conditions could be simultaneously detected by mass spectrometric assays but only those findings that trigger an immediate therapeutic or dietary intervention are actually communicated to the parents and the attending pediatrician.

Eventually, and that has been a major obstacle for many recent developments, the measurement of new diagnostic parameters must also be feasible in a routine environment, that is, in a robust, standardized, and quality-controlled fashion generating sufficiently precise and accurate data that warrant the expected sensitivity and specificity (or rather, *in praxi*, positive and negative predictive values) [9, 10]. Of course, all of the above has to be achieved keeping the commercial viability in mind, that is, balancing the disease-related socio-economic impact and the savings made possible by refined disease management against the actual costs of the new diagnostic tools.

2. The rationale for new diagnostic markers

2.1. Unmet medical need and socio-economic impact

For chronic kidney disease (CKD), a thorough assessment of the aforementioned aspects is rather straightforward although many epidemiological and economic figures have an unexpectedly large uncertainty in the relevant literature. Chronic kidney disease (listed in chapter N18 of the International Classification of Diseases—ICD10) has a very high—and almost certainly underestimated—prevalence in the general population; most recently published figures range from 5 to 7% in global evaluations [11–13], to roughly 8–10% for the adult population in Western countries [14, 15]. More specialized studies also claim markedly higher numbers, for example, 16.8% in the National Health and Nutrition Examination Survey (NHANES) of the adult Americans [16, 17]. Most of these differences are clearly caused by discrepant diagnostic criteria and definitions, on which the statistics in the reports are based (e.g. proteinuria AND/OR pathologically low estimated glomerular filtration rate (eGFR) vs. impaired eGFR alone). Whatever the actual prevalence of a defined diagnostic finding in a certain population may be, there is a pronounced age-dependency (8.5% in 20–39-year-old people, 12.6% in 40–59-year-old, and 39.4% in >60 year-old, respectively [16, 17]) and a moderate but still highly significant ethnic difference (19.9% in black vs. 16.1% in white Americans of non-Hispanic origin; $p < 0.0001$). Obviously, though, the strongest associations exist with the most relevant etiologies: diabetes and hypertension, which, together, cause approximately 75% of all cases of CKD (40.2% in diabetics vs. 15.4% in euglycemic individuals; 24.6% in hypertensive patients vs. 12.5% in normotensive individuals; both $p < 0.0001$) (**Figure 1**).

In all of these analyses, the most worrying observation is that the demographic changes and the presently much-discussed pandemic of obesity, type II diabetes mellitus (T2D) and other Western lifestyle-associated diseases will further increase these figures (particularly in developing countries). In fact, epidemiological surveys already identify these changes in the weight of the different etiologies: the percentage of type II diabetics among patients initiating renal replacement therapy has more than doubled in the last two decades [18]. Many experts stress the obvious pathophysiological relevance of a high-salt diet for CKD via hypertension; however, high sodium intake also seems to be an independent risk factor both for poor therapeutic efficacy of anti-hypertensive treatment with angiotensin converting enzyme (ACE) inhibitors and for rapid progression to end-stage renal disease (ESRD) [19].

Chronic kidney disease is responsible for an alarming number of deaths, but these numbers may still be underestimated because the mortality is more often due to comorbidities and sequelae, particularly cardiovascular disease (CVD) and its clinical endpoints myocardial infarction (MI) and stroke, or to complications of renal replacement therapies, than to kidney failure itself. Throughout the mass of publications on cardiovascular complications in CKD and the causal relationships (lately summarized by Alani et al. [20]), the broad consensus is that CKD patients are much more susceptible to CVD, particularly to coronary artery disease (CAD); in fact, after age-adjustment, CKD patients have a 15- to 30-times higher risk to die of CVD than the general population [21, 22], and in ESRD patients, all-cause mortality is 10- to 100-times elevated compared to individuals with normal renal function [23].

It may be very difficult if not impossible to completely unravel the chicken and egg problem of whether kidney damage is causing CVD or vice versa, even if the study design is diligently targeting this question and sophisticated statistical tools are applied to correct for all potential confounders. The most plausible interpretation is that both conditions have common pathomechanisms, for example, inflammation, oxidative stress, and endothelial dysfunction, and so they frequently co-develop. At any rate, the huge socio-economic burden caused by the network of obesity, hypertension, diabetes, CKD, and CVD can hardly be overrated. In

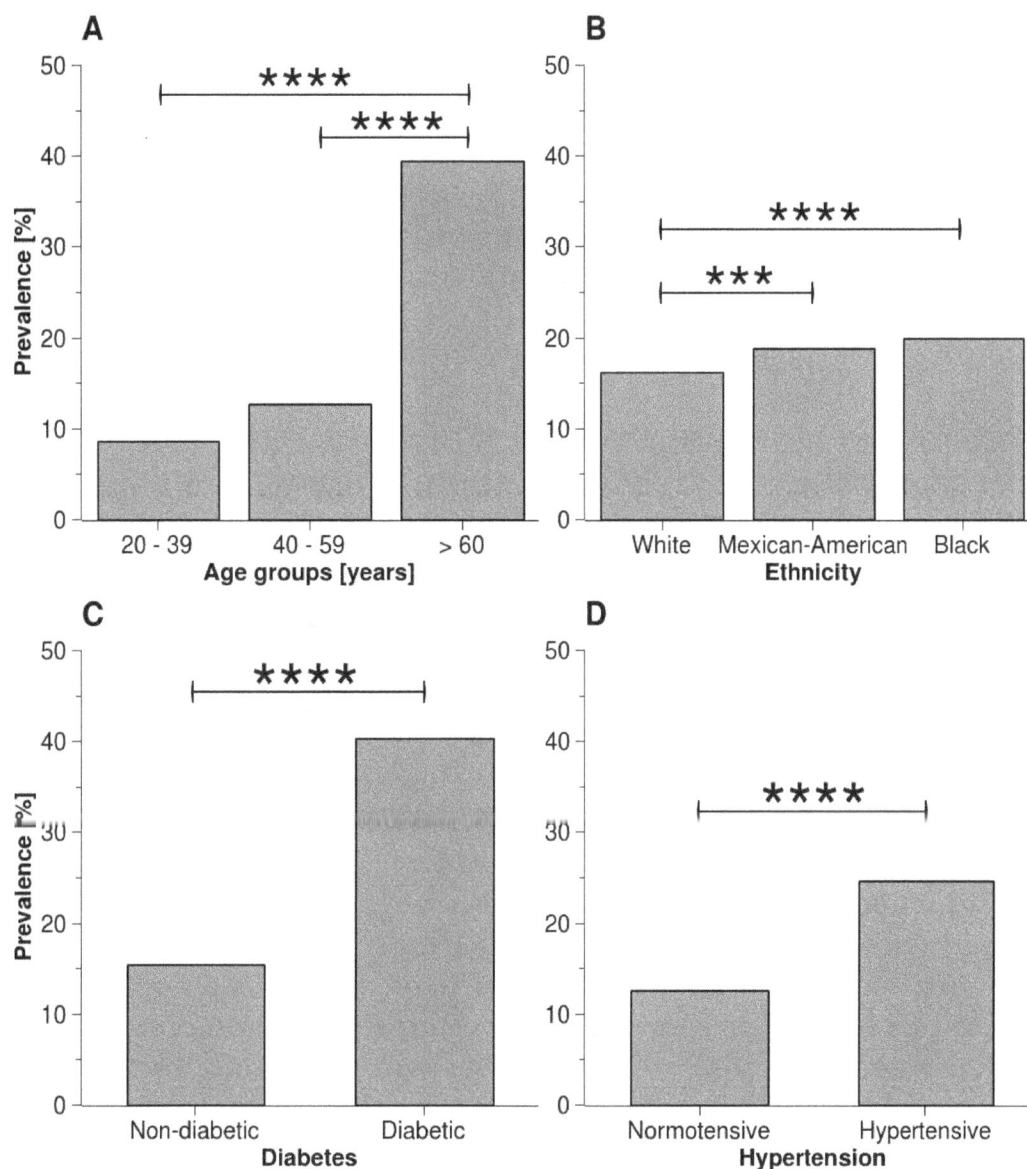

Figure 1. Prevalence of CKD among adults in the USA [16, 17]. (A) Age-related increase: 8.5% in the third and fourth decade, 12.6% in the fifth and sixth, and 39.4% in individuals more than 60 years old. (B) Ethnic background: 16.1% in white Americans (non-hispanic), 18.7% in Mexican-Americans (p < 0.001), and 19.9% in black Americans (p < 0.0001). (C) Etiology, role of glycemic control: 40.2% in diabetic patients vs. 15.4% in non-diabetics; p < 0.0001. (D) Etiology, role blood pressure: 24.6% in hypertensive patients vs. 12.5% in normotensives; p < 0.0001. *** p < 0.001 **** p < 0.0001. Modified after [82].

terms of global mortality, these non-communicable conditions have long exceeded the most problematic infections, and the pivotal role of CKD in this closely interwoven network has recently been dissected in a truly compelling paper [23].

As noted above, the spending for renal replacement therapy (RRT, be it hemodialysis or transplantation) is disproportionately high; in industrialized countries, as much as 2–3% of the entire health care budget can go into treatment of ESRD patients [24]. A more specific calculation published by the United States Medicare system demonstrates that 18.2% of the total budget are necessary for the 9.2% of recipients who are CKD patients (any stage in this statistics), and this discrepancy is aggravating at an alarming rate: in the last decade, CKD-related costs have surged almost four times faster than the overall Medicare expenditures (380 vs. 100% increase; United States Renal Data System [25]). Moreover, there is no doubt that this situation will further worsen because ESRD is still a globally undertreated condition. In the near future, much more than the approximately 2–3 million ESRD patients who are currently receiving RRT [26] will have access to appropriate treatment, particularly in developing countries where 1 million people are estimated to die from untreated ESRD each year [27].

2.2. Shortcomings of available diagnostic tools

The second major motivation for exploring new diagnostic biomarkers for CKD is the extremely poor performance of the currently available parameters. There is a considerable number of publications and probably just as much clinical hearsay around this issue, so that even a somewhat comprehensive treatise cannot fit here. Still, a couple of concise problems related to the estimated glomerular filtration rate (eGFR), the most frequently used basis for diagnosing, staging, and monitoring CKD, shall be discussed:

First and most obvious, the eGFR is only a calculated estimate of a very informative but, *in praxi*, difficult-to-obtain gold standard parameter describing kidney function—the experimentally measured glomerular filtration rate (mGFR). Despite huge efforts to optimize approximations such as the Cockcroft-Gault (CG), the Modification of Diet in Renal Disease (MDRD), and—more recently—the Chronic Kidney Disease Epidemiology Collaboration (CKD-EPI) equation for adults, or the Counahan-Barratt for pediatric patients [28–31], these estimates have a common weakness since they are all based on creatinine levels, which are themselves influenced by anthropometric variables like muscle mass, and whose increase under pathophysiological conditions may be blunted by higher rates of creatinine secretion in the proximal tubule. In any case, they all have important flaws that are of the utmost clinical relevance [32–34].

More specifically, while all of the aforementioned formulas seem to work reasonably well in large cohorts, that is, a statistical assessment will yield acceptable correlation coefficients, the estimates for an individual at a given time can differ from the actual mGFR to a drastic degree. Extremely problematic examples have been reported where patients with an mGFR of zero had eGFR values of 40–50 ml/min/1.73 m^2 (i.e. stage III CKD according to the recommendations of the Kidney Disease Outcomes Quality Initiative, KDOQI), thus severely underdiagnosing a life-threatening condition [35]. On the other hand, it is generally acknowledged that the approximations perform particularly poorly and tend to underestimate the actual kidney function at higher, near-healthy levels of glomerular filtration rate (GFR) (>60 ml/min/1.73 m^2) [36]. This shortcoming was implicitly accepted when developing the CG and MDRD equations; the CKD-EPI development, in contrast, specifically included healthy cohorts but the formula still does not perform well enough in some of the most common and clinically relevant situations for assessing renal function, for example, for patients to be given contrast agents in radiology who have kidney-related risk factors or potential donors for organ transplantation *inter vivos*. Both indications specifically rely on accurate estimates in the near-normal range. The catastrophic failure of all current equations to meet this expectation was recently highlighted in a compelling analysis [37]: in a study comprising almost 300 potential living kidney donors, eGFR values below 80 ml/min/1.73 m² (the typical cut-off for acceptance of living donors) had positive predictive values (PPV) for an mGFR below this threshold of only 0–40% with the vast majority of situations (formula, age, sex, and BMI) yielding less than 20% (**Figure 2**). In other words, many—actually most (!)—potential donors would have been declined on the basis of a falsely low eGFR, which cannot be justified considering the dramatic shortage of donor organs in general [38] and the much better clinical outcome of donations *inter vivos* compared to *post mortem* [39, 40].

2.3. Therapeutic consequences?!

As noted in the introduction, decision-makers in diagnostics companies, in insurances, and in clinical practice will scrutinize new biomarkers or assays regarding their actual diagnostic performance but also regarding the clinical utility of the additional information they provide, that is, their therapeutic consequences. Of course, such deliberations can always be countered by the thought-terminating cliché that better diagnostic tools will eventually facilitate better standards of care for patients or, in this concise case, earlier diagnosis of impaired renal function and more accurate staging/monitoring of CKD will allow for more informed clinical

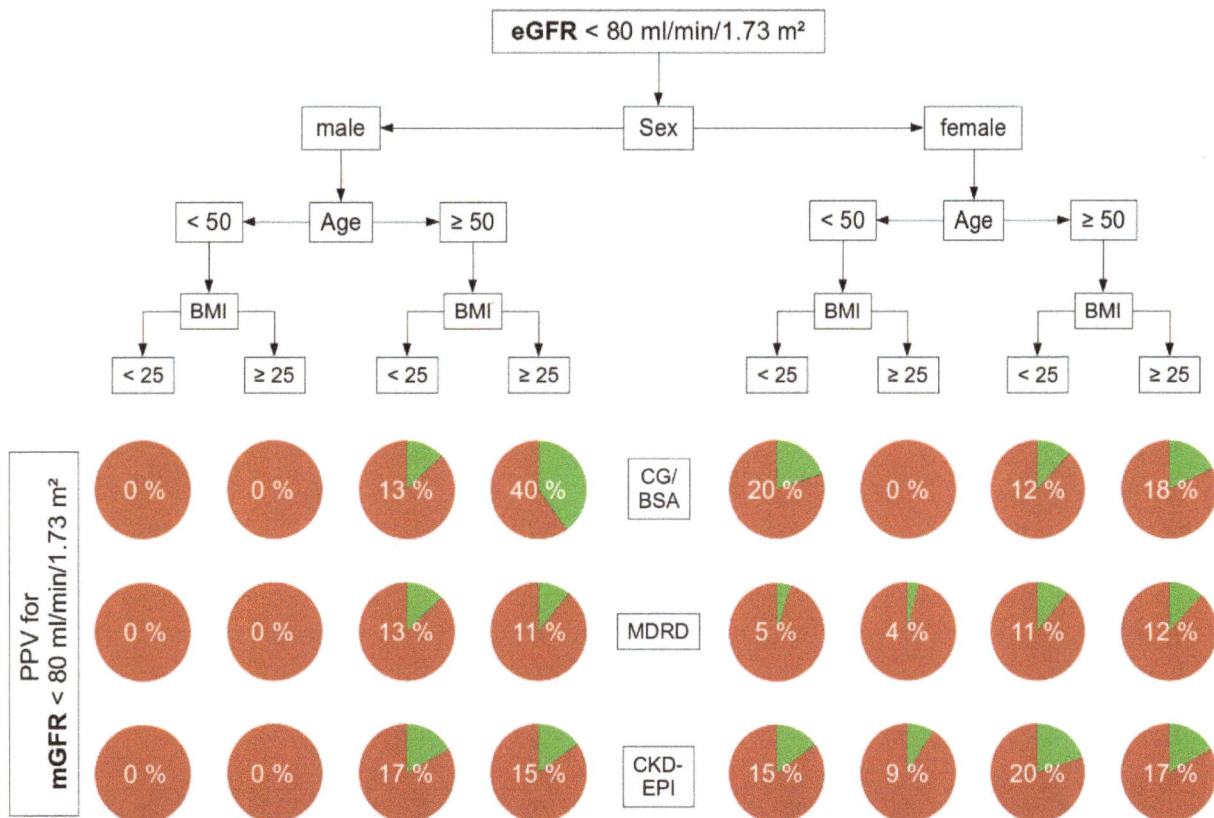

Figure 2. Limited diagnostic reliability of eGFR in the near-normal range. Positive predictive values (PPVs) for a measured GFR below 80 ml/min/1.73 m² in individuals with an eGFR below 80 ml/min/1.73 m², modified after [37, 82]. Subsets are analyzed according to sex (male vs. female), age (<50 vs. >50) and BMI (<25 vs. >25). Estimates of GFR are calculated using any of the three most common equations: Cockcroft-Gault per body surface area (CG/BSA), modification of diet in renal disease (MDRD), or chronic kidney disease epidemiology collaboration (CKD-EPI). All PPVs are below 40%, in most cases even below 20%.

decisions, thus more effective disease management, and a slower progression of patients to ESRD. Yet, the evidence for such generic and ambitious claims was quite sparse until, around the end of the last century, rather aggressive treatment regimens were tested in long-term, controlled studies.

These recent developments, however, define a surprisingly clear rationale for diagnostic innovation in this field: first, precise and accurate evaluation of renal function in (practically) healthy individuals gains in clinical relevance, that is, with glomerular filtration rates in the (almost) normal range, for which the commonly applied equations have exceptionally poor positive predictive values (for a detailed example, see Section 2.2, **Figure 2**).

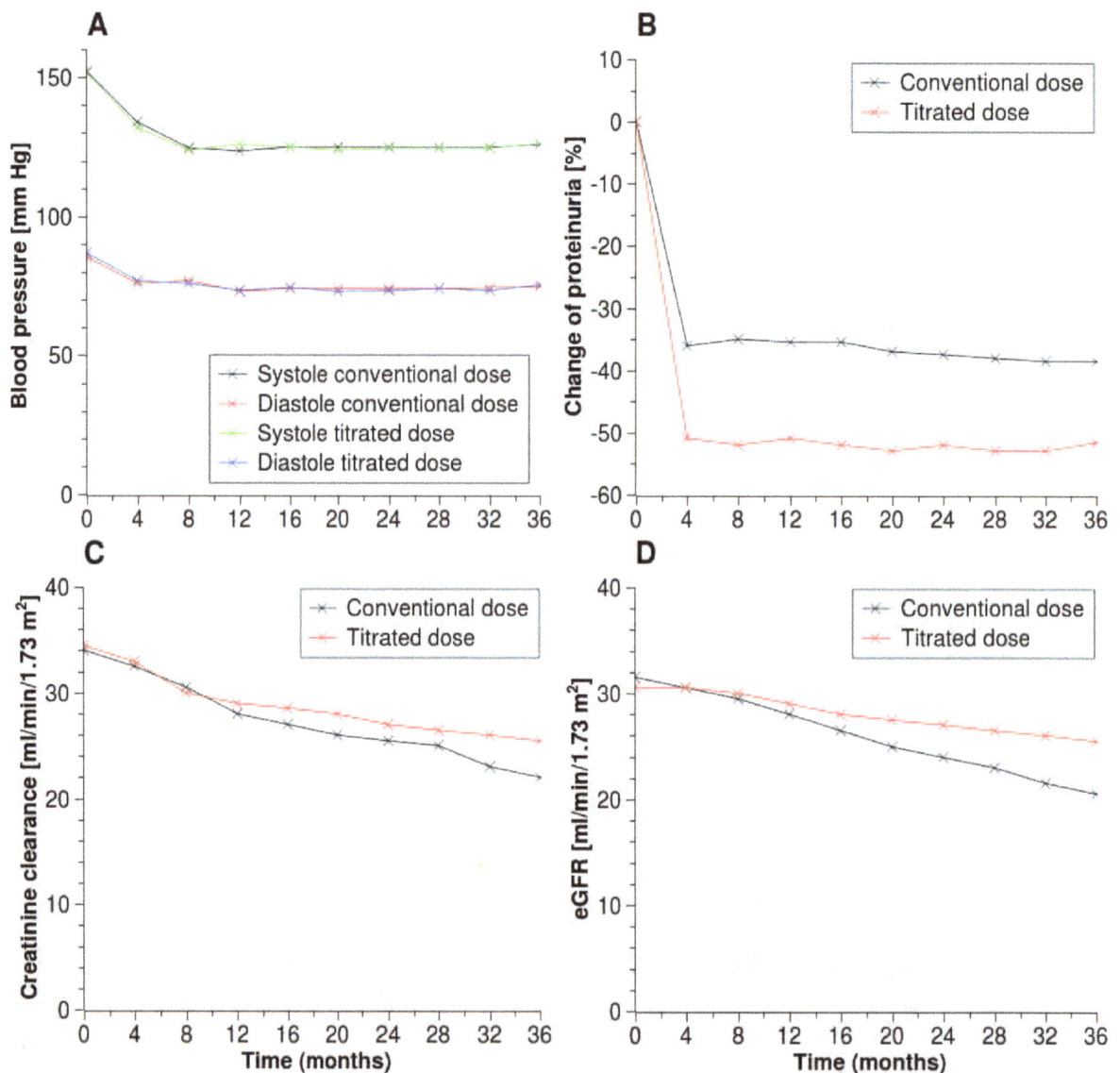

Figure 3. Efficacy of aggressive therapeutic regimens. Data from the Renoprotection of Optimal Antiproteinuric Doses (ROAD) study, modified after [41, 82]. (A) Maximizing the antiproteinuric effect by increasing the doses of benazepril and losartan (within tolerated limits) in euglycemic CKD patients did not further lower the blood pressure but (B) improved albuminuria markedly more than the conventional dose and significantly postponed the decline of (C) creatinine clearance and (D) eGFR during a 3-year follow-up period.

Second, the therapeutic approaches available for CKD patients have been revolutionized in the last 20 years, and the significant benefits of personalized, multi-modal, and titrated regimens have been demonstrated beyond any doubt. The Renoprotection of Optimal Antiproteinuric Doses (ROAD) study clearly showed that maximizing the antiproteinuric effect by up-titration of ACE inhibitors (e.g. Benazepril™) and Angiotensine-II-Receptor-Subtype-1 (AT1) antagonists (in this case, Losartan™) to individually tolerated limits in euglycemic CKD patients did not further lower the blood pressure in comparison to standard treatment but was far superior in reducing albuminuria and in delaying the decrease of eGFR and creatinine clearance in a 36-months follow-up [41] (**Figure 3**). Maybe even more impressive, the so-called 'Remission Clinic' program initiated at the Istituto Mario Negri in Milan, a staggered intervention strategy consisting of a low-sodium and low-protein diet with an ATI antagonist, an ACE inhibitor, a calcium channel blocker, and a statin—each in titrated doses—could drastically reduce the incidence of ESRD in a 7-year observation period. Concisely, in two paired cohorts consisting of 56 individuals each, 17 patients (30.4%) who received the standard treatment developed ESRD but only 2 (3.6%) who were treated according to the Remission Clinic protocol did so, which translated into an odds ratio for progressing to ESRD of only 0.092 under the more aggressive treatment scheme [42, 43].

3. Biomarker discovery for CKD

The motives examined in Section 2 have spurred significant efforts in all modern disciplines of bioanalytics—genomics, transcriptomics, proteomics, and metabolomics—aiming at the identification and validation of new biomarkers or biomarker panels addressing the unmet diagnostic needs and overcoming the flaws of the currently available solutions.

In genomics, genome-wide association studies (GWAS) have identified a large number of single nucleotide polymorphisms (SNP) significantly associated with the risk of developing CKD, incident diabetic nephropathy, renal function, and metabolic traits associated with CKD [44–52], and these findings already shed new light on pathomechanisms and regulatory networks in CKD although they seem to be quite far from routine clinical applications (see below).

Expression profiling of messenger ribonucleic acid (mRNA) and micro ribonucleic acid (µRNA) species found patterns associated with the risk of disease progression [53], the repair of acute kidney injury [54], various etiologies of CKD [55], the role and function of the immune system before and during hemodialysis [56], and with the regulation of atherogenic pathways in CKD [57].

Based on top-down and bottom-up proteomics workflows, a range of new kidney-related biomarkers have been advocated, for example, kidney injury molecule 1 (KIM-1), neutrophil gelatinase-associated lipocalin (NGAL), fibroblast growth factor 23 (FGF-23), monocyte chemotactic protein 1 (MCP-1), or urine retinol-binding protein 4 (uRBP4) [58, 59]. In addition, there is particularly vivid research on urinary peptides; most of these peptides are products of the turn-over of the extracellular matrix and, actually, derived from collagen ([60]; Mischak, personal communication). Over more than a decade, a compelling body of data has been accumulated documenting a clinically relevant diagnostic and prognostic performance of one particular panel of urinary peptides called CKD273 [61–65].

Chronic kidney disease and related indications such as nephrotoxicity also range among the most frequently addressed subjects in metabolomics, partly because of their clinical, societal, and commercial impact (see above), partly also because—from a purely scientific angle—they are considered to be rather straightforward targets or even 'low-hanging fruits'. It is perfectly reasonable to believe that a functional impairment of organs with such a central role in metabolism as the kidneys will alter the systemic homeostasis to a degree that should be easily detectable in blood or urine by state-of-the-art bioanalytics. The same reasoning led metabolomics towards some of its greatest successes so far, for example, the much more detailed characterization of the pathobiochemistry of type II diabetes, the evidence-based assessment of anti-diabetic drugs in preclinical and clinical development, and even the identification of highly promising and biochemically plausible biomarker signatures for the early diagnosis of prediabetes/impaired glucose tolerance and for an individual risk assessment as much as a decade before the manifestation of the disease [9, 66–70]. Even more disruptive, an utterly compelling proof-of-concept for the utility of mass spectrometry (MS) as a diagnostic tool was achieved by implementing routine screening programs for many genetically determined metabolic defects, the so-called 'inborn errors of metabolism', based on quantitative multiplex assays for amino acids and acylcarnitines [71, 72]. Originating from pilot projects in the mid-1990s, this screening is now available in most industrialized and several developing countries and clearly set the stage for the workflow that is today called targeted metabolomics [9, 73, 74].

4. Metabolic biomarker candidates for CKD

The sizeable number of publications on kidney-related metabolomics studies mentioned above— and there may be a comparable amount of work performed by the pharmaceutical industry that has not been published—suggest an immense array of potential metabolic biomarker candidates. Over the last few years, several teams of experts went to great lengths to summarize these results in very systematic review articles [59, 75–77]. This chapter, however, follows a slightly different and maybe less comprehensive but hopefully complementary approach by highlighting alterations in selected metabolic pathways instead of individual molecules. Also, it focuses on findings that fulfill additional quality criteria, that is, for which there is relevant translational evidence, quality-controlled quantitative data, and at least some degree of mechanistic plausibility.

Of course, when claiming mechanistic insights based on typical metabolomics studies, one must never ignore the fact that anabolic and catabolic pathways are not the only factors influencing the homeostatic concentrations of metabolites in urine or peripheral blood. Nutritional uptake, microbial metabolism in the gastro-intestinal tract and urinary excretion (and, of course, hemodialysis in ESRD patients!) play equally fundamental roles. Unfortunately, in the large population-based studies, these aspects are never documented in sufficient detail and reliability to be suitable for a quantitative assessment (e.g. questionnaire-based reports on nutritional habits [78]). So, in a way, the pathway-centric methodology used in this chapter can only reflect one set of possible explanations for how metabolite concentrations are altered, and this shortcoming is primarily caused by difficult-to-avoid gaps in the documentation of most biomarker studies. Yet, the clinical experience from screening millions of newborns demonstrates that this particular limitation can be partly overcome: as soon as ratios of products and substrates of enzymatic reactions (or entire pathways) are analyzed instead of individual metabolite concentrations, the data are far less prone to all sorts of confounding factors such as dietary uptake and rather reflect the actual metabolic activity of the organism [66, 79–81].

4.1. Creatinine

At first sight, it is hardly worth mentioning that the most frequently found metabolite indicative of CKD is creatinine [15, 82]. However, this simple statement has two fundamentally different reasons: First and quite trivial, creatinine is indeed a marker for kidney function and has rightly been established as one of the most common diagnostic parameters for many years although—as noted above—its performance (both as a single laboratory parameter and as the basis for calculating the eGFR) is far from perfect.

Second, and this must be kept in mind for all further considerations: the vast majority of all studies in this field enrolled and staged or classified patients according to their eGFR and, thus, indirectly also according to their creatinine levels. Therefore, identifying creatinine as a statistically significant marker metabolite is just a typical case of self-fulfilling prophecy (it is actually quite revealing that, in many cases, creatinine does NOT rank as the top candidate, that is, does not have the highest significance level or the lowest p-value).

On the other hand, what is the alternative? Due to obvious cost, time, and compliance issues, the number of studies that are based on mGFR or hard clinical endpoints is rather limited, and so the subsequent discussion does not exclude eGFR-based studies as a matter of principle but instead tries to substantiate the level of confidence in the various findings through a synopsis of statistics (significance, independent replication), translational research (relevance of models and match of patterns in different species), and biochemical scrutiny (pathway mapping, enrichment analyses, or similar approaches).

4.2. Dimethylarginine metabolism

Considering all single metabolic markers and/or panels that have been suggested so far, the most compelling preclinical and clinical evidence underpins a central role of dimethylarginine metabolism and, in particular, of symmetric dimethylarginine (SDMA) [83–85].

A quick look at the underlying biochemistry: the guanidinium side chains of arginine residues in polypeptides are the targets for specific post-translational modifications by a set of isoenzymes called protein arginine N-methyltransferases (PRMT), which are evolutionarily well conserved from unicellular eukaryotes such as yeast all the way to humans [86]. In two consecutive reactions, first monomethylarginine and then one of the two possible isomers of dimethylarginine are formed: an asymmetrically substituted version (ADMA) if one ω-nitrogen atom carries both methyl groups, and a symmetric version (SDMA) in case the methyl groups are bound to both terminal nitrogens (**Figure 4**).

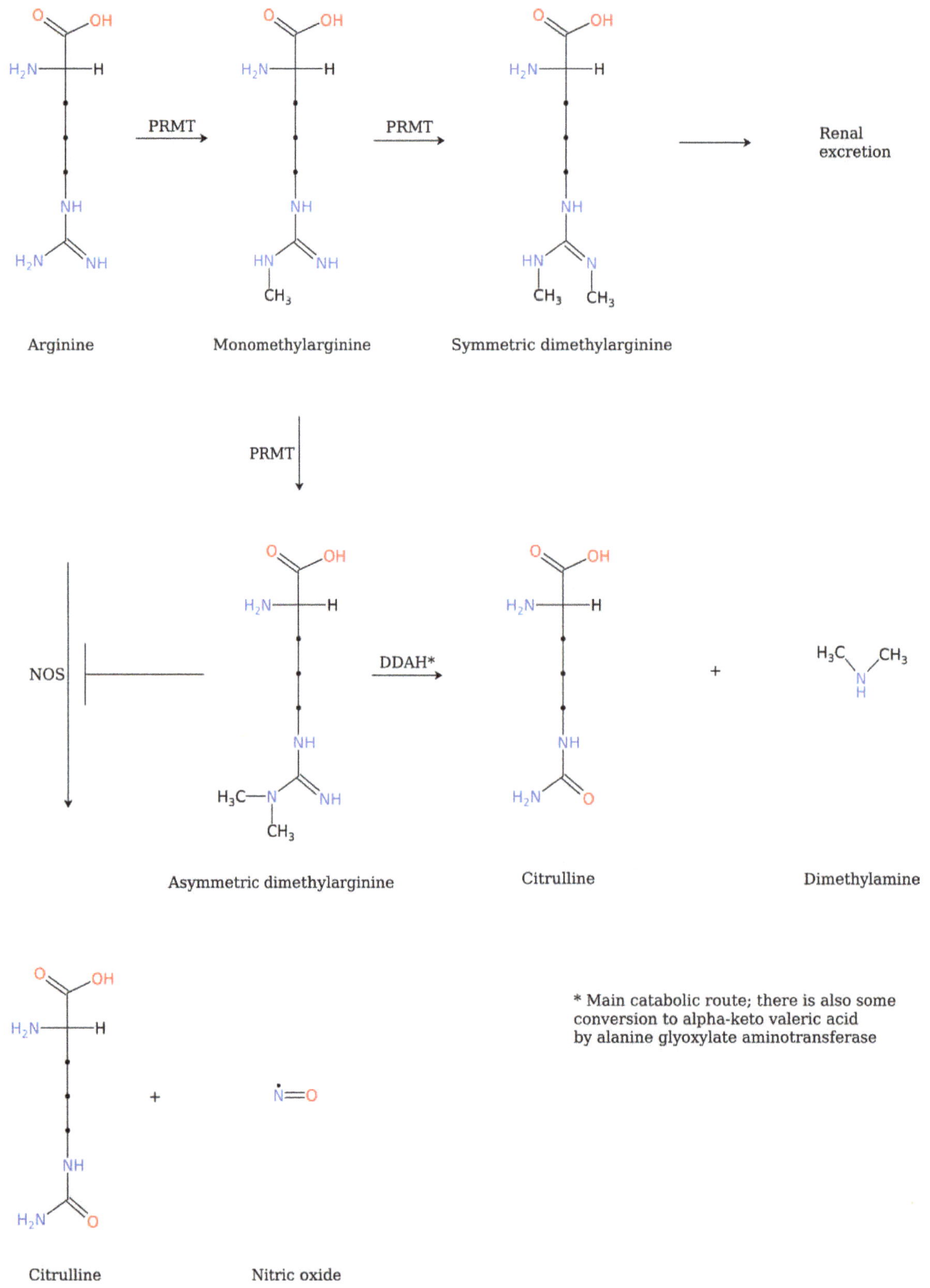

Figure 4. Metabolism of dimethylarginines. Schematic summary of dimethylarginine metabolism (modified after [82]). In two subsequent reactions, arginine sidechains are mono- and then dimethylated resulting in either asymmetric (ADMA) or symmetric dimethylarginine (SDMA). ADMA is a potent inhibitor of nitric oxide synthases (NOS), which produce nitric oxide (NO) through direct conversion of arginine to citrulline, and is mainly metabolized to citrulline and dimethylamine. In contrast, SDMA is metabolically inert and primarily eliminated via the kidneys.

Although these two molecular species are structurally quite similar (isomers, in fact), their physiological roles differ quite fundamentally. To be more specific, ADMA acts as a potent endogenous inhibitor of nitric oxide synthases (NOS) and, therefore, high concentrations lead to a decreased systemic production of nitric oxide (NO). Thus, ADMA is promoting or aggravating endothelial dysfunction, and elevated levels of ADMA may be among the functionally most meaningful cardiovascular risk factors in general [87, 88]. Once released by proteolysis, the bulk of ADMA is catabolized to citrulline and dimethylamine by two isoforms of dimethylarginine dimethylaminohydrolase (DDAH) while SDMA is biologically rather inert, hardly metabolized in the body and, instead, eliminated via the kidneys.

In widely used animal models of kidney injury such as Sprague-Dawley rats treated with the nephrotoxic aminonucleoside antibiotic puromycin, SDMA levels in plasma were shown to increase in a dose- and time-dependent manner [89, 90] (**Figure 5A**). A very similar correlation was observed in a cross-sectional study on CKD patients; both in diabetic nephropathy and in non-diabetic CKD (mainly hypertensive patients), later stages of the disease were characterized by significantly higher concentrations of SDMA in plasma, further corroborating that the observed changes are linked to the severity of kidney damage instead of the underlying etiology [89, 91] (**Figure 5B**). The statistical significance of this finding was even stronger when using the SDMA-to-Arginine ratio (corrected analysis of variance (ANOVA) p-value in the range of 10^{-11} instead of 10^{-9} for SDMA alone [82]) although this is not a simple product-to-substrate ratio as briefly discussed above [66]. For a more detailed discussion of the outstanding improvements that a systematic exploration of such metabolite ratios can achieve both in statistical power and in biological plausibility, please refer to recent genome-wide association studies on phenotypes defined by targeted metabolomics, the first highly synergistic combination of different omics platforms to date [81, 92, 93].

Quite incomprehensibly, several current review articles on metabolic biomarkers for kidney failure do not even mention SDMA [15, 76] although the scientific and clinical evidence underpinning its diagnostic potential is undeniable. A thorough meta-analysis of 20 clinical studies encompassing more than 2100 patients demonstrated beyond any reasonable doubt that there is a highly significant association of SDMA and creatinine concentrations on the one hand, and an inverse correlation of SDMA levels and several measures of renal clearance on the other [94]. Admittedly, in some of these studies, ADMA was also identified as a marker candidate, describing markedly elevated levels in individuals with impaired kidney function [84, 91, 94]. However, this must be seen as part of the aforementioned chicken and egg problem: CKD and cardiovascular disease are very closely interwoven and, therefore, alterations of both conditions' most significant biomarkers will frequently coincide. Yet, there is a relatively simple but revealing clinical observation that plausibly links ADMA to cardiovascular risk and SDMA to kidney function: after kidney transplantation, ESRD patients have at least partially restored renal function, and their SDMA levels drop quickly and markedly while, at the same time, ADMA concentrations stay elevated [95].

4.3. Tryptophan metabolism

The second group of CKD-associated metabolic changes to be discussed here is substantiated by especially convincing evidence from translational research: tryptophan metabolism. Tryptophan

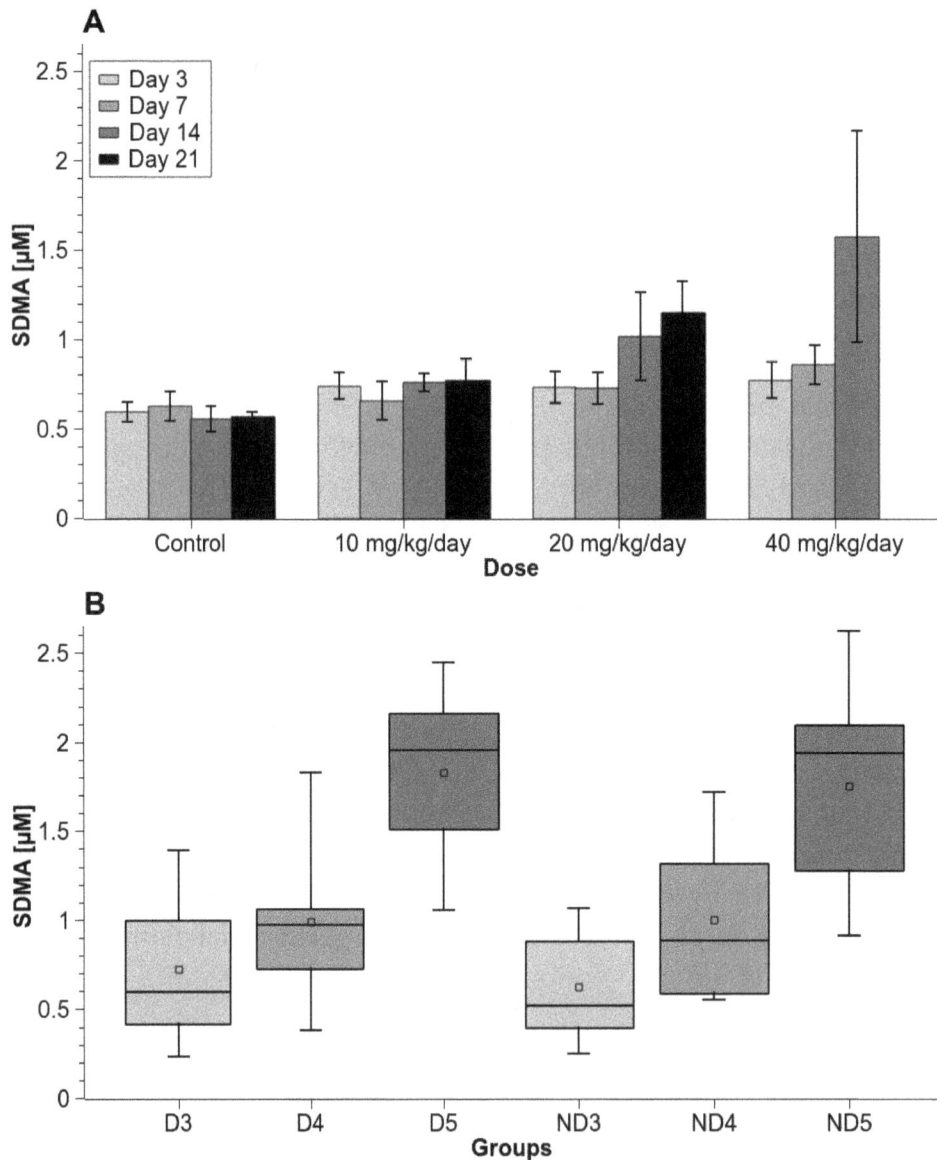

Figure 5. SDMA in translational research. (A) Puromycin-induced renal impairment in Sprague-Dawley rats [89, 90]. Plasma SDMA concentrations show a dose- and time-dependent increase. For the group receiving the highest dose, the last time-point is missing; due to complete renal failure, these animals had to be sacrificed before day 21. (B) UroSysteOmics study: in a cross-sectional analysis of CKD patients, both diabetic (D) and non-diabetic (ND) individuals had significantly elevated plasma SDMA levels at later stages of their kidney disease (p-values for all pairwise comparisons of clinical stages 3, 4, and 5: $p(D3/D4) = 0.18$, $p(D4/D5) = 2.7 \times 10^{-3}$, $p(D3/D5) = 7.83 \times 10^{-5}$, $p(ND3/ND4) = 0.11$, $p(ND4/ND5) = 9.8 \times 10^{-3}$, $p(ND3/ND5) = 3.8 \times 10^{-4}$). Modified after [82, 89, 91, 113].

is a non-polar, aromatic amino acid, has the bulkiest sidechain in the proteinogenic repertoire, is essential in humans, and has long been the subject of particular interest for neurobiologists because it is the starting point for the biosynthesis of the neurohormone melatonin [96] and the neurotransmitter serotonin [97]. Lately, though, the alternative catabolic pathway originating from tryptophan, the kynurenine pathway, which ultimately leads to niacin via quinolinate, has drawn much more attention because of the immunomodulatory and tolerogenic effects [98–100] of the enzyme catalyzing the rate-limiting step in this pathway, indoleamine-2,3-dioxygenase, which oxidizes tryptophan to N-formyl-kynurenine [101, 102] (**Figure 6**).

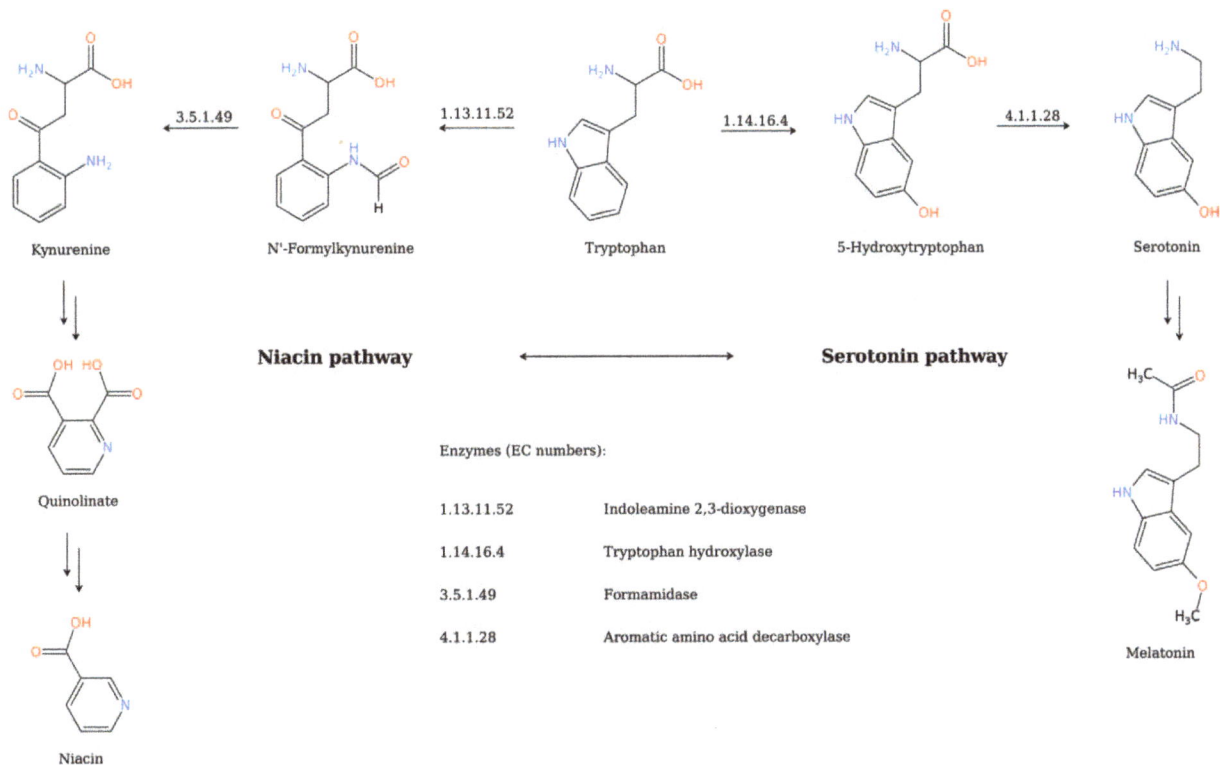

Enzymes (EC numbers):	
1.13.11.52	Indoleamine 2,3-dioxygenase
1.14.16.4	Tryptophan hydroxylase
3.5.1.49	Formamidase
4.1.1.28	Aromatic amino acid decarboxylase

Figure 6. Tryptophan metabolism. Schematic summary of tryptophan catabolism (modified after [82]. The essential amino acid tryptophan is the substrate for two different pathways, the so-called serotonin pathway producing the neurotransmitter serotonin [97] and the neurohormone melatonin [96], and the so-called kynurenine pathway leading to the synthesis of niacin via its precursor quinolinate.

Increased turn-over of tryptophan in animal models with renal insufficiency has been observed as early as the 1960s, for example, in spontaneously hypertensive rats [103], and tryptophan depletion in peripheral blood has been identified in different sorts of nephropathies [104, 105], although these studies relied on a rather limited analytical armamentarium. Yet, these very early observations have recently been confirmed in two independent animal models, namely in Sprague-Dawley rats treated either with adenine or puromycin to induce kidney damage. In fact, two completely different workflows led to the same conclusions: Untargeted metabolic profiling of serum, urine, and kidney tissue identified tryptophan as a biomarker candidate distinguishing adenine-treated rats from untreated controls [106, 107] and, based on a targeted and analytically validated quantitative data set, the aforementioned puromycin model had already shown the same effect [89, 90]. The latter study, due to its longitudinal design with three dose escalation arms, could demonstrate very clearly that, upon puromycin treatment, plasma tryptophan concentrations decreased in a dose- and time-dependent manner (**Figure 7A**) and, even more notable, they plunged to below one-third of the baseline levels observed in the group receiving a vehicle-only control. Effect sizes of this magnitude may be quite frequently found in urine (or in other omics disciplines, for that matter) but they are almost unheard of in plasma or serum where the homeostatic regulation of all amino acid concentrations is typically very stringent—even under rather drastic environmental conditions, various dietary influences, exhausting physical exercise, or pharmacological interventions [9, 66, 78, 108–112].

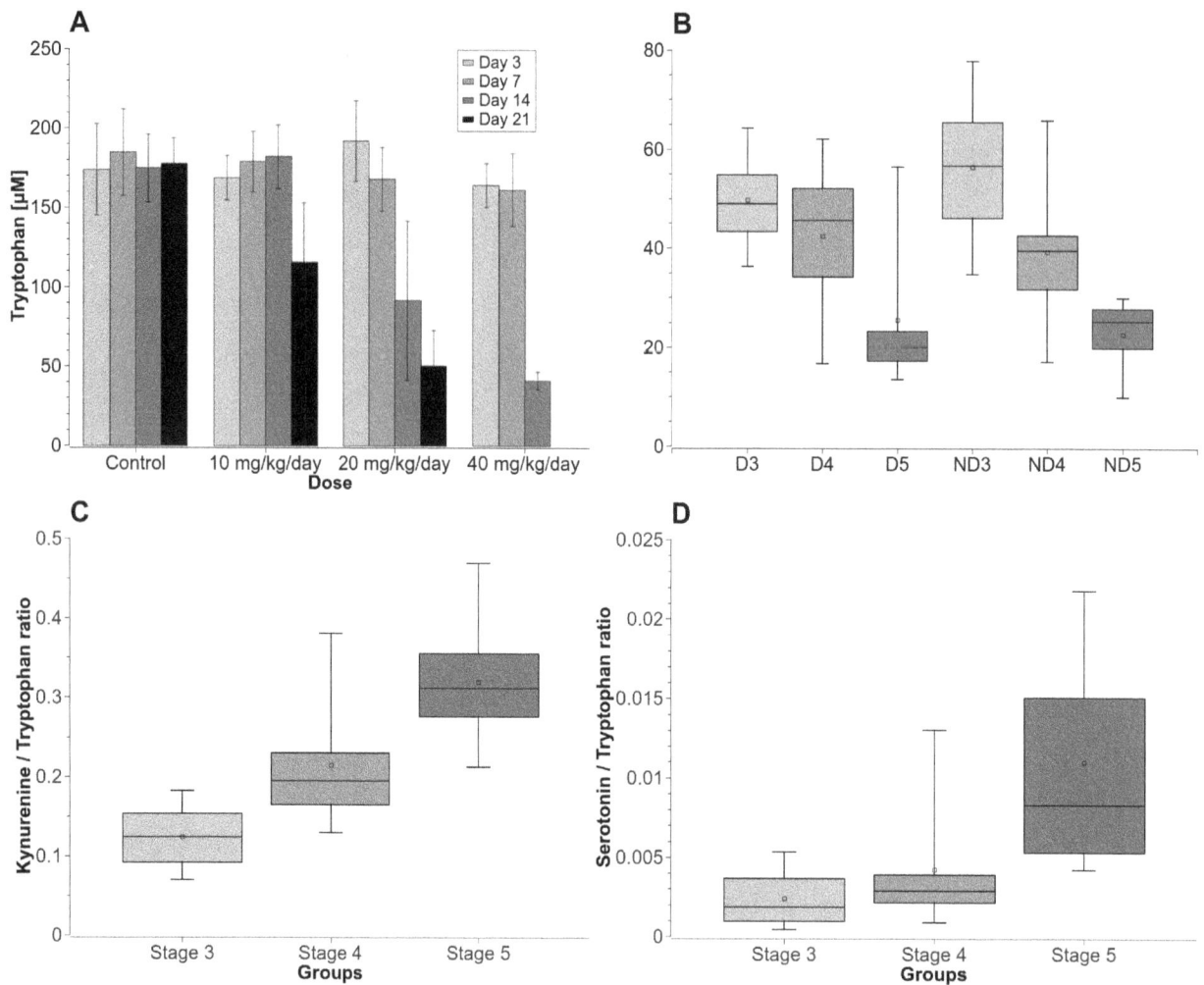

Figure 7. Tryptophan in translational research. (A) Puromycin-induced kidney injury in Sprague-Dawley rats is accompanied by dramatically decreasing plasma tryptophan concentrations, and this effect is both dose- and time-dependent [89, 90]. (B) Cross-sectional analysis of diabetic and non-diabetic CKD patients (UroSysteOmics study [89, 91, 113, 114]): independent of the underlying etiology, median tryptophan levels in stage 5 are less than half of the values in stage 3 (p-values for all pairwise comparisons of clinical stages 3, 4, and 5: $p(D3/D4) = 0.47$, $p(D4/D5) = 2.3 \times 10^{-3}$, $p(D3/D5) = 3.89 \times 10^{-4}$, $p(ND3/ND4) = 0.041$, $p(ND4/ND5) = 2.50 \times 10^{-3}$, $p(ND3/ND5) = 2.12 \times 10^{-6}$). (C) The kynurenine-to-tryptophan ratio, indicative of the activity of the kynurenine pathway, is markedly higher in later stages of CKD [$p(stage3/stage5) = 1.44 \times 10^{-12}$]. (D) The serotonin-to-tryptophan ratio, indicative of the activity of the serotonin pathway, is markedly higher in later stages of CKD [$p(stage3/stage5) = 2.98 \times 10^{-6}$]. Modified after [82].

As shown for dimethylarginine metabolism (see Section 4.2), these alterations in tryptophan metabolism are also very convincingly replicated by translational research. In this case, both cross-sectional studies on specifically selected patients [89, 91, 113, 114] and larger population-based cohorts [115, 116] were able to demonstrate that tryptophan concentrations in serum and plasma are significantly lower in patients with less residual kidney function, that is, at a later stage of CKD (**Figure 7B**). Just as in the animal models described above, the absolute magnitude of this depletion is quite remarkable: the median tryptophan levels in stage 5 patients are more than 50% lower than in stage 3 patients, and these drastic changes seem largely independent of the underlying etiology as indicated by a separate subgroup analysis of diabetic and non-diabetic patients (**Figure 7B**).

It has been known for a very long time—more than half a century—that tryptophan is specifically bound and transported by albumin (elucidated in impressive physico-chemical detail by McMenamy and Oncley [117]), and more recent publications estimate that 75–90% of the circulating tryptophan is actually present in a bound form [118, 119]. The continuous excretion, that is, loss, of albumin in proteinuric animals and patients could, thus, influence these findings in a highly relevant manner (considering the relatively low binding affinity—depending on the experimental conditions, the apparent association constant k' is approximately 10^4—and the absolute concentrations reported, it is fair to assume that the assays used were measuring total instead of free tryptophan although neither publication directly comments on this question). A quantitative comparison of data from the UroSysteOmics study, however, sheds some light on these speculations: the drop of the tryptophan levels is much more pronounced than that of the albumin concentrations in the same period (−58 vs. −19% from stage 3 to stage 5 [89]), so it is evident that there must be other mechanisms involved in depleting tryptophan than just a loss of transport capacity.

Indeed, both aforementioned pathways metabolizing tryptophan appear to be dramatically upregulated in later stages of CKD as underpinned by significantly elevated ratios of serotonin and kynurenine to tryptophan, respectively [89, 91, 113, 114] (**Figure 7C** and **D**). In a large independent study, the kynurenine-to-tryptophan ratio was one of the strongest predictors of changes in kidney function between consecutive visits of study subjects in the Cooperative Health Research in the Region of Augsburg (KORA) S4 and F4 surveys and also of newly diagnosed CKD in this roughly 7-year period [115]. Besides these extremely convincing findings with significant diagnostic and prognostic potential, tryptophan plays yet another, albeit less direct role in CKD: it is the starting point for the synthesis of indoxyl sulfate (IS), one of the most intensely discussed and, arguably, also most dangerous uremic toxins. Some of the dietary tryptophan (as noted, Trp is an essential amino acid in humans) is cleaved to indole by the gut microbiota. Indole is absorbed by the intestinal mucosa and, ultimately, metabolized to IS in hepatocytes [120]. In an impressive number of reports, IS has been characterized as a nephrovascular toxin [121], an indicator of poor residual renal function [122], and a prognostic biomarker predicting elevated risks for vascular disease and all-cause mortality in CKD patients [120].

Of course, cleaving indole from Trp is only one of the countless ways, in which the gut microbiome may affect the pathophysiology of CKD and, more specifically, the systemic availability of many metabolites. The multifaceted connection between the microbiota and CKD—too complex to be discussed here—has recently been reviewed in great detail and, notably, also examined for its potential as a target for specific therapeutic interventions [123].

4.4. Urea cycle alterations, nitric oxide synthesis, and polyamine metabolism

A less straightforward and sometimes even controversial set of observations presents itself around another well-known pathway, the urea cycle and its interfaces with nitric oxide synthesis and polyamine metabolism (**Figure 8**). More concisely, a longitudinal analysis of a fairly large subset of the KORA cohort (more than a thousand individuals), identified spermidine as one of the biomarker candidates with the best statistical significance [115]; it was inversely correlated with the annual eGFR change, especially in people without a diagnosis of CKD at baseline, which clearly confirmed findings from the early 1980s [124, 125]. Yet, quite surprisingly, some of the most recent reviews on biomarkers in nephrology do not even mention spermidine at all [59, 75, 76].

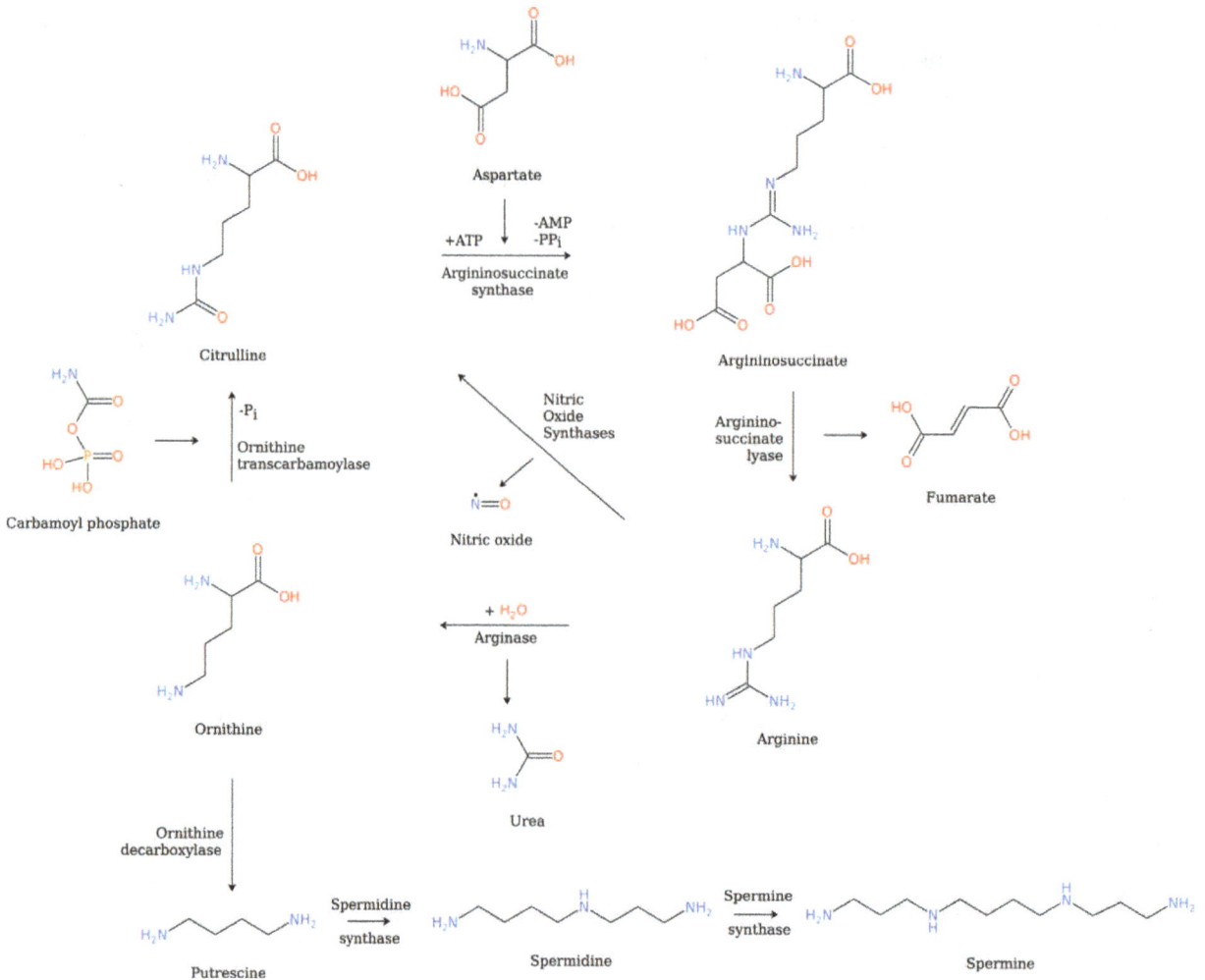

Figure 8. Urea cycle, nitric oxide and polyamine production. Schematic summary of the urea cycle and its connections to polyamine and NO production. As discussed in Section 4.4., the levels of biomarker candidates such as arginine, ornithine, and citrulline are regulated in a complex manner; therefore, interpretation of the data for this pathway is quite speculative, except for spermidine, which is only involved in polyamine synthesis. Modified after [82].

In the UroSysteOmics patients, citrulline-to-arginine ratio was significantly higher at later stages of CKD ($p = 3.5 \times 10^{-3}$ for diabetics, $p = 3.7 \times 10^{-3}$ for non-diabetics). In theory, this could, of course, be caused by a higher activity of nitric oxide synthases (although this is quite unlikely in a situation of pronounced oxidative stress; see Section 4.5) just as well as from a combined effect of arginase and ornithine transcarbamoylase (OTC) activities in the urea cycle. A more detailed evaluation showed that there were etiology-specific differences in this pathway: in euglycemic patients, ornithine-to-arginine ratio was markedly higher at later stages of CKD ($p = 7.8 \times 10^{-5}$) while, in diabetic patients, this ratio was not associated with the degree of renal failure in a significant manner [89, 91, 113]. Further mechanistic studies are certainly required to untangle the intricacies of these observations because arginase also plays a role in the regulation of NO synthesis and vascular function beyond just competing with NOS for their joint substrate, arginine [126].

Considering the pathogenetic relevance of endothelial dysfunction and the well-documented NO deficiency in CKD (reviewed by Baylis [127]), it is—again—quite surprising that arginine, ornithine, and citrulline have so far hardly been discussed as biomarker candidates [15, 128, 129]. This may either mirror gaps in the analytical portfolio—after all, metabolomics is not a comprehensive omics discipline yet, and even less so if studies are based on a single technology or workflow—or a lack of pathway-oriented data analysis [79, 80].

4.5. Oxidative stress and functional consequences

With 16,605 PubMed-listed publications in 2017 alone, oxidative stress, that is, a biochemical imbalance of oxidizing and reducing agents but most often just referring to reactive oxygen species and their detoxification, is clearly one of the most intensely studied concepts of pathobiochemistry, and probably even of modern biology in general. In fact, looking at the literature, it seems that there is hardly a disease, in which oxidative stress is not one of the major culprits. Its pivotal role in CKD has been identified and reviewed hundreds of times from the 1980s to the present [130–134], so—for completeness' sake—it must be discussed here, too. Although there is a very broad agreement in the community about the finding itself and its clinical relevance, no direct diagnostic application of that knowledge has been achieved so far, mainly for (pre-)analytical reasons. Oxidative stress causes damage to various groups of biomolecules such as amino acids, lipids, or nucleotides by processes that are extremely well understood on the molecular level [135–138]. However, these reactions often generate quite unstable intermediates, for example, peroxides of unsaturated fatty acids (**Figure 9**). Therefore, fragments from the cleavage of such oxidized lipids (usually malone dialdehyde and 4-hydroxynonenal) are commonly detected as surrogate markers. Other compounds require tricky preanalytical procedures or challenging analytical methods, for example, nitrated amino acids or oxidized nucleotides. Highly sophisticated sample preparation protocols and mass spectrometric assays have been developed for many of these analytes [139, 140] but, due to their complexity and limited robustness, they are still far from a routine application in clinical chemistry.

A rather stable and analytically more accessible measure of oxidative stress was recently suggested and already applied in several studies, namely methionine sulfoxide and its ratio to unmodified methionine [108, 111, 113, 141, 142]. Methionine sulfoxidation is a posttranslational modification (PTM) of methionine residues caused by various oxidizing agents, for example, hydrogen peroxide, hydroxyl radicals, hypochlorite, chloramines, and peroxynitrite, and has frequently been reported to cause a more or less severe loss of function in modified proteins [143].

As may have been expected, the patients enrolled in the UroSysteOmics study had markedly higher methionine sulfoxide-to-methionine ratio, the more advanced their CKD became, and that could be observed in diabetic and non-diabetic patients in a very similar fashion [89, 91, 113]; (**Figure 10**). Interestingly, the broad coverage of the targeted metabolomics experiments combined with hypothesis-driven data analytics and interpretation allowed to corroborate this finding by depicting functional consequences of the oxidative conditions in the same data set. Under oxidative stress, the activities of enzymes that depend on oxidation-sensitive cofactors, for example, tetrahydrobiopterin (BH4), have been reported to drop due to a limited availability of these cofactors [144–147]. In principle, this applies to NOS but, in practical terms, the effect on the citrulline-to-arginine ratio is often masked by alterations in the urea cycle as discussed above (Section 4.4). In the present case, the activity of phenylalanine hydroxylase (PAH) was a much more plausible read-out parameter. When a relevant percentage of BH4, an essential cofactor for PAH, is oxidized to 4-α-hydroxytetrahydrobiopterin, it is no longer

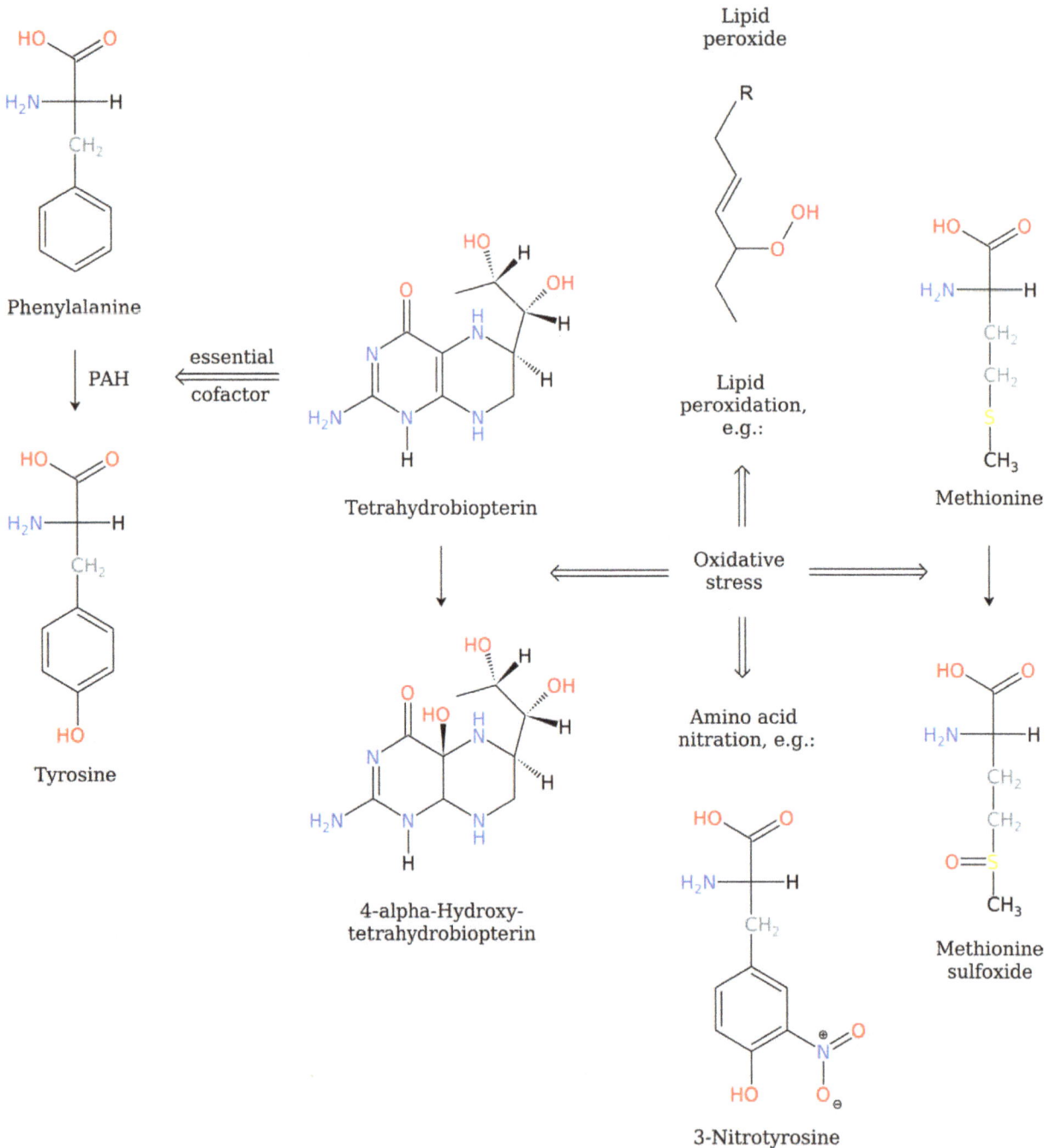

Figure 9. Oxidative stress. Simplified overview of some biochemical consequences of oxidative stress (modified after [82]). Unbalanced oxidative conditions cause chemical modifications to various classes of metabolites, for example, lipid peroxidation, amino acid nitration, or oxidation of nucleotides. Many products of these reactions are very unstable or — for other reasons — difficult to analyze, therefore, the methionine-sulfoxide-to-methionine ratio is now commonly used as a robust surrogate for these parameters. In the same context, highly reduced cofactors, for example, tetrahydrobiopterin, are oxidized and — thus — no longer sufficiently available to warrant a normal level of enzymatic activity. In the example chosen here, this affects the enzyme catalyzing the first step in phenylalanine catabolism, phenylalanine hydroxylase, which leads to a 'phenylketonuria-like' phenotype characterized by a lowered tyrosine-to-phenylalanine ratio.

available in sufficient quantities to ensure normal PAH activity and, so, one observes a 'phenyl-ketonuria-like' phenotype with a decreased tyrosine-to-phenylalanine ratio (**Figure 9**). In fact, these opposing trends could be clearly observed in the quantitative data: just as methionine sulfoxidation rates increased from moderate to severe disease in the UroSysteOmics cohort, the PAH ratio continuously dropped towards later stages of CKD, and this was again independent of the underlying etiologies [89, 91, 113] (**Figure 10**). In very good accordance with this finding, the cross-sectional analysis of the KORA F4 cohort revealed a strong and highly significant negative correlation of phenylalanine levels with eGFR (effect size: 2.36 ml/min/1.73 m^2 per SD, p = 7.8 × 10^{-22}). One has to concede that this correlation was not significant in a replication cohort (UK Twins), possibly because of the much smaller sample size, but the pooled analysis of both cohorts still yielded a rather convincing p-value of 1.4 × 10^{-18} [116].

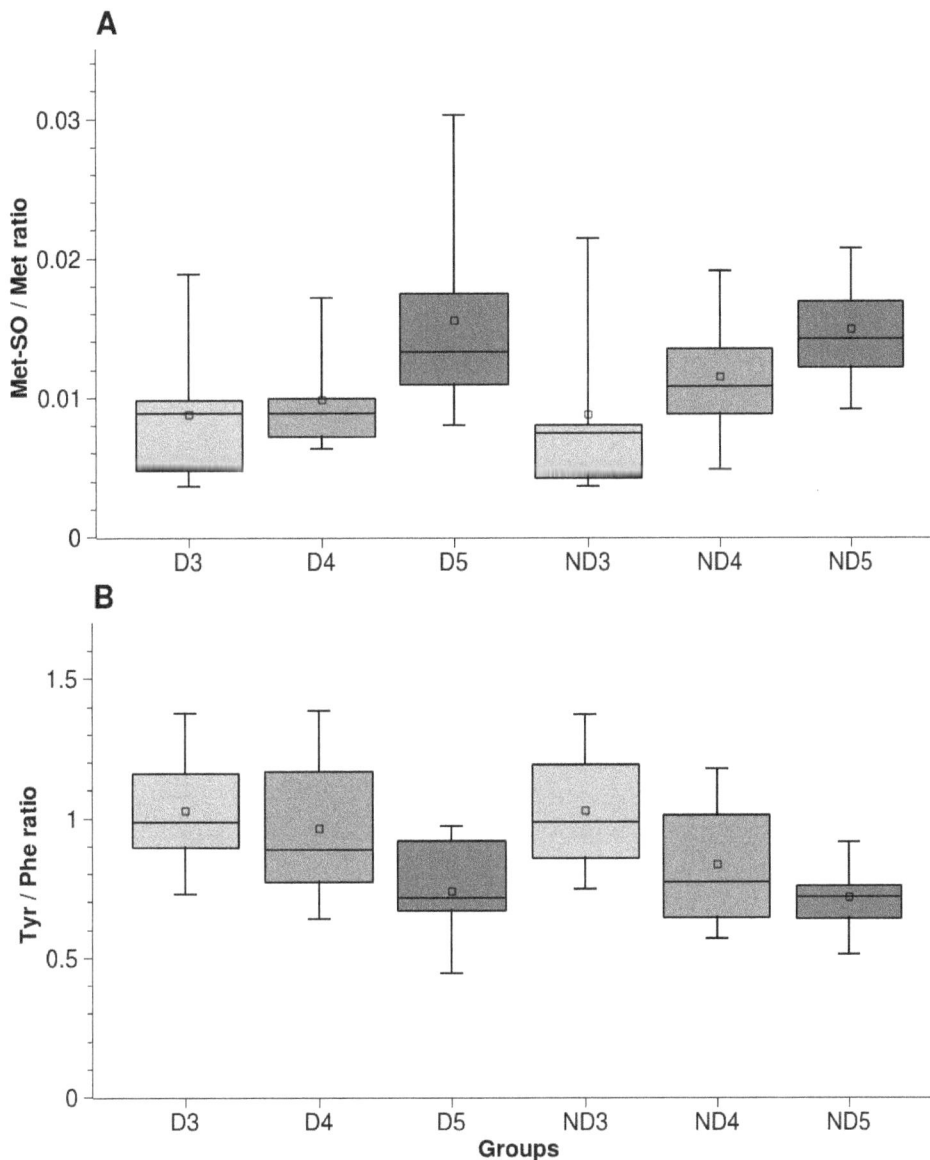

Figure 10. Oxidative stress and its functional consequences in CKD. Data from the UroSysteOmics cohort [89, 91, 113] demonstrating the parallel increase of methionine sulfoxidation and impairment of phenylalanine hydroxylase. (A) Significantly elevated ratios of methionine sulfoxide to methionine at advanced stages of CKD, observed both in diabetic and non-diabetic patients (p-values for all pairwise comparisons of clinical stages 3, 4, and 5: p(D3/D4) = 5.49 × 10^{-3}, p(D4/D5) = 0.024, p(D3/D5) = 4.22 × 10^{-4}, p(ND3/ND4) = 3.7 × 10^{-3}, p(ND4/ND5) = 0.088, p(ND3/ND5) = 4.21 × 10^{-5}). (B) Decreased activity of phenylalanine hydroxylase in patients with more advanced disease as demonstrated by lower tyrosine-to-phenylalanine ratio, also hardly influenced by the status of the glycemic control (p-values for all pairwise comparisons of clinical stages 3, 4, and 5: p(D3/D4) = 0.68, p(D4/D5) = 0.12, p(D3/D5) = 0.023, p(ND3/ND4) = 0.12, p(ND4/ND5) = 0.18, p(ND3/ND5) = 0.015). Modified after [82].

4.6. Acylcarnitines

Particularly strong alterations in nephrology-related metabolomics studies were observed in a class of compounds that does not get much attention in mainstream biochemistry but has been part of the standard diagnostic repertoire since the beginning of the mass spectrometry-based era in newborn screening [71, 72], the acylcarnitines. Long-chain fatty acids are the primary substrates for β-oxidation in the mitochondria and, thus, one of the pivotal energy sources in the cell. Yet, they can neither cross the double membrane of the mitochondria as free fatty acids nor as fatty acyl esters of coenzyme A (CoA), which is their metabolically activated form. Instead, tissue-specific isoforms of carnitine palmitoyl transferase I (CPT-I) located at the outer mitochondrial membrane first trans-esterify the fatty acyl residues from CoA to carnitine, a quaternary ammonium compound derived from lysine. The resulting acylcarnitines are then taken across the inner membrane by an antiporter system named carnitine acylcarnitine translocase (CACT). On the matrix face of the inner membrane, a second carnitine palmitoyl transferase (CPT-II) re-esterifies the fatty acids to CoA, and this fatty acyl-CoA can then undergo p-oxidation while the released carnitine is returned to the cytoplasm to be available as a carrier again (a cyclic process thus called the carnitine shuttle) [148–150].

In the aforementioned study on puromycin-induced nephrotoxicity in rats, the plasma levels of acylcarnitines of various chain lengths surged in a dose- and time-dependent manner [82, 89, 90], and this may be understood as a consequence of increased mitochondrial leakage caused by apoptosis or other sorts of damage to the mitochondrial membranes (a basal level of leakage must be assumed to explain the fact that acylcarnitines are detectable in peripheral blood at all).

As for the marker candidates discussed previously, there is striking translational evidence supporting these findings both from population-based and from smaller, dedicated clinical studies. In a cross-sectional assessment of the KORA F4 data, 26 acylcarnitines showed statistically significant correlations with renal function, that is, eGFR, with the strongest effect size of 3.74 ml/min/1.73 m^2 per SD and a compelling p-value of 2.2×10^{-52} for glutarylcarnitine, and most of these hits were confirmed as significant in the UK Twins cohort [116]. Also in the UroSysteOmics study, certain species of acylcarnitines such as glutarylcarnitine (C5-DC) or pelargonylcarnitine (C9) showed significantly elevated levels in patients with more advanced kidney disease, again independent of the etiology (ANOVA p-values for the trend across stages 3, 4, and 5 of 3.9×10^{-6}, 1.7×10^{-4}, 3.4×10^{-4}, and 4.4×10^{-5} for C5-DC and C9 in diabetics and non-diabetics, respectively) [89, 113].

One has to consider, however, that many of these acylcarnitines have very low absolute concentrations in healthy or early stage patients (typically in the low nanomolar range) and, so, many individual values that were the basis of the statistical evaluation may have been around or even below the lower level of quantitation (LLOQ) of the assays applied in these studies (Biocrates Absolute*IDQ* P150 and P180 kits [151, 152]). Of course, this does not necessarily put the observation itself into question (since these kits were real first-in-class products, the LLOQ values were chosen very conservatively; in the validation and in routine applications, the precision was still extremely good at the lower end of the calibration curves; and, finally, even the qualitative difference of a marker being below LLOQ at early stages and well above at later stages could bear meaningful diagnostic information) but some of the published significance levels could be slightly overestimated.

All of the above leaves one important question to be discussed: three independent clinical cohorts ranging from population-based to specifically selected in the clinics identify C5-DC as the most significant marker candidate in this class of metabolites—is there any plausible mechanistic explanation for this particular finding? Glutaric acid (systematically: pentanedioic acid) is an intermediate of lysine, hydroxylysine, and tryptophan catabolism, and elevated concentrations are the eponymous hallmarks of glutaric acidemias, autosomal recessive deficiencies of various enzymes affecting this pathway [153, 154]. Yet, besides some observations that neonates with glutaric acidemias can sometimes also have birth defects like polycystic kidneys, there is no convincing genetic or metabolic link in the literature between glutaryl-CoA dehydrogenase and CKD, for example, a higher rate of heterozygotes among patients with renal failure or the like. However, the explanation may also be much easier: C5-DC as a dicarboxylic compound could simply be a product of ω-oxidation of fatty acids, that is, a side effect of the oxidative stress discussed in Section 4.5.

4.7. Other potential biomarkers

In addition to the aforementioned, a plethora of other metabolites has been suggested as potential biomarker candidates in sample types like serum, plasma, urine, or even feces [15]. These include (without any claim of completeness): nucleosides and nucleotides (1-methylinosine, 1-methyladenosine, adenine, adenosine, 2-deoxyadenosine, guanine, hypoxanthine, inosine, thymidine, and xanthosine), amino acids and biogenic amines (alanine, aspartate, betaine, carnosine, choline, glutamate, glycine, homocystine, hypotaurine, indoxyl sulfate, isoleucine, leucine, proline, taurine, trimethylamine-N-oxide, and valine), vitamin derivatives (5C-aglycone), intermediates of the citric acid cycle (α-ketoglutarate, fumarate, and isocitrate) and other organic acids (acetate, adipate, citrate, galactarate, hippurate, lactate, maleate, malonate, methyl-malonate, pantothenate, pyruvate, and azelate), bile acids (chenodeoxycholic acid), carbohydrates (glucose, maltose, myo-inositol), and various lipids either found in specialized lipidomics studies or as part of broader metabolomics approaches (polyunsaturated fatty acids like docosapentaenoic and docosahexaenoic acid, but also dihydrosphingosine, phytosphingosine, and several lysophosphatidylcholines) [82, 89, 113, 114, 128, 155–173].

As noted, this list is certainly not exhaustive and primarily presents compounds that were identified in clinical samples, but it may also highlight that these biomarker candidates range from well-known uremic toxins like indoxyl sulfate to xenobiotics like azelate, the role of which can only be subject to speculation.

On the other hand, many of these metabolites may just represent typical confounders, for example, reflect characteristics of the underlying etiology of CKD or comorbidities such as diabetes [174]: pyruvate and glucogenic amino acids like alanine, serine, and glycine, for instance, directly mirror the systemic glycolytic or gluconeogenic flux; glycolysis replenishes their pools while gluconeogenesis tends to deplete them [9, 66]. Also closely linked to diabetes are the branched-chain amino acids (BCAA): leucine, isoleucine, and valine accumulate in peripheral blood in a situation that bears a striking resemblance to insulin resistance [9, 66, 175], and they are—particularly in combination with the aromatic amino acids (AAA)—some of the earliest predictors of incident type II diabetes [68].

Similarly, lysophospholipid levels (and, even more so, their ratios to intact phospholipids) are directly correlated to the activity of phospholipases, which represents the first step in a cascade that releases various polyunsaturated fatty acids (PUFA) from membrane phospholipids and, eventually, produces oxidized PUFA-derivatives such as prostaglandins, leukotrienes, thromboxanes, and others, thus mirroring the systemic level of inflammation rather than an organ-specific effect [176–178].

In conclusion, a very long list of metabolic changes has been identified in individuals with impaired renal function and in relevant animal models of kidney damage. However, from a diagnostic point-of-view, it seems that only a limited subset of these marker candidates has been underpinned by quality-controlled quantitative data [9, 10, 108] analyzed by appropriate bioinformatics strategies [79, 179–182], diligent study design that allows for an assessment of the specificity of the observations, and mechanistic insights based on translational research and a detailed biochemical understanding of the differentially regulated pathways [66, 79, 80, 182]. Yet, the marker candidates fulfilling these criteria could certainly have a significant potential in clinical chemistry, particularly if they are (or have been) successfully replicated in independent clinical cohorts [116] and scrutinized in studies specifically designed to test their prognostic value [115, 183, 184].

5. Multiparametric metabolic biomarker panels

Up to now, the majority of studies in this field have analyzed their data sets to identify single metabolites as candidate biomarkers but, as noted above, derived parameters such as ratios of product and substrate concentrations of a particular enzymatic reaction or an entire metabolic pathway, are extremely powerful tools for finding correlations with larger effect sizes, better statistical significances, and, notably, also higher biochemical plausibility [9, 66, 71, 72, 79–81, 92, 116, 175, 182]. Yet, and that was one of the basic assumptions nurturing the immense optimism at the beginning of the omics era in biomedical research and development, the superior information content offered by the comprehensive analytical platforms could only be harnessed by using broader, multiparametric panels or even signatures as biomarkers. To this end, two profoundly different strategies for defining such panels have been successfully applied in CKD-related metabolomics, one guided by biochemical background knowledge and the other by hypothesis-free bioinformatics approaches.

5.1. Knowledge-based biomarker panels

Hypothesis-driven attempts to define multiparametric diagnostic signatures are founded on a detailed, pathway-oriented description and—whenever possible—also a mechanistic understanding of the pathobiochemical changes identified in particular studies [79, 80]. If specific sets of such metabolic alterations are repeatedly observed, for example, the various effects discussed in Section 4, it would seem logical and straightforward to devise simple linear combinations of concentrations or ratios to refine the diagnostic performance. To illustrate this point, here is one very simplistic example based on the UroSysteOmics data set (not an optimized model that, of course, cannot be revealed in this context): Various versions of generic scores like this (Eq. (1)) easily outperformed the individual ratios; this was demonstrated by relevant improvements of the area under the receiver-operating-characteristics curve (AUROC) for the distinction of stage 4 from stage 3 (in the combined cohort, i.e., irrespective of the etiology) from 0.75 to 0.853 [114], and these equations can and, in fact, must be extended and further optimized for each diagnostic indication. However, in contrast to early hopes in theoretical biology, this strategy does not work *ad infinitum*. The area under the curve (AUC) does not asymptotically converge to 1.0 if one only adds enough parameters with the intention to 'exhaustively' describe the biological system (more is not always better). In most cases (unfortunately, as with so many important aspects of metabolomics, there are hardly any relevant publications on this subject), the AUC peaks for signatures comprising 5–20 metabolites and then drops again, supposedly because more features add too much analytical and biological 'noise'. In one concise example, for which this was analyzed in a systematic fashion, panels of plasmalogens were checked for their performance in the (admittedly trivial) distinction between diabetics and euglycemic controls. Plasmalogens are phospholipids that have one fatty acid linked to the polar head group by an ester bond and the second residue by an enol ether bond, whose concentrations continuously drop during the progression of the metabolic syndrome towards manifest type II diabetes. Starting with the single most significant molecular species and then adding up to six plasmalogens in a linear combination as shown in Eq. (1) improved the AUC from 0.92 to 0.95 but further addition of up to 35 features from the same class caused the AUC to drop to 0.88, that is, below the value for the best monoparametric marker [10, 79, 182].

$$S = a\frac{[SDMA]}{[Arg]} + b\frac{[Kyn]}{[Trp]} + c\frac{[Met - SO]}{[Met]} \tag{1}$$

Such 'constructed' marker panels are transparent, plausible, even intuitively pleasing and, thus, have a reasonable likelihood of gaining acceptance in the clinical community, they certainly fail to take advantage of the entire information content of a given data set in a systematically optimized way. Therefore, the definition of marker panels and the generation of diagnostic/prognostic algorithms are increasingly based on hypothesis-free strategies such as machine learning, network analysis, and other advanced data mining strategies.

5.2. Panel selection and optimization by machine learning

In contrast to the hypothesis-driven definition of metabolic biomarker panels described above, a much more technical selection process can be conducted by means of machine learning. The roots of machine learning as a discipline promoted by a rather special community date back to the middle of the twentieth century, when the legendary Alan Turing published his groundbreaking work on 'Computing machinery and intelligence' [185]. Still in the 1950s, the 'Dartmouth summer research project on artificial intelligence' took place as a kick-off meeting for the entire field [186], Arthur Samuel presented his seminal paper 'Some studies in machine learning using the game of checkers' [187] and Ray Solomonoff first discussed his idea on 'An inductive inference machine' which he later extended and matured in his 'Theory of inductive inference' [188].

Machine learning is closely related to the fields of artificial intelligence (AI), knowledge discovery, and data mining. It investigates systems and algorithms that learn from experience (data) to improve its performance, and is traditionally split into three major arms: supervised, unsupervised, and reinforcement learning. The main objective in supervised learning is the recognition of patterns or the predictive classification (e.g. the distinction of cases and controls in a clinical trial) by approaches such as k-Nearest Neighbor (kNN) classification, Bayesian networks, logistic regression, decision tree learning, support vector machines (SVMs), or neural networks. In contrast, unsupervised learning applies a descriptive approach to detect unknown patterns and rules in data sets, to cluster data, or to identify classes, which were not previously defined, for example, by using partitioning-based approaches such as k-means clustering, density-based strategies, or hierarchical clustering. The third variety, reinforcement learning, uses the principle of cumulative rewards to optimize the actions of a software agent in complex situations [189–191].

Successful attempts to define biomarker panels by machine learning were recently conducted based on the metabolomics and proteomics data sets from the UroSysteOmics study [183]. In a rather typical workflow, potential biomarker candidates were initially identified by univariate statistics of differences between groups of patients with early and advanced stages of CKD. Multiparametric classifiers were then developed by supervised machine learning using support vector machines (SVM) [192]. To this end, 76 putative biomarkers, which showed statistically significant differences between the defined cohorts, were combined into 3 distinct panels: 'MetaboP' consisting of 17 plasma metabolites, 'MetaboU' comprising 13 metabolites in identified in urine, and finally 'Pept' consisting of 46 urinary peptides (for the far more advanced panel CKD273 consisting of urinary peptides analyzed on the same platform, see Section 3). The performance of these three classifiers was evaluated in an independent test set by checking their correlations with renal function (eGFR) at baseline and at a follow-up visit approximately 2 years later. Each of the classifiers showed a very good correlation with baseline eGFR, that is, in a diagnostic setting, but—much more excitingly—also with the renal function at the follow-up examination indicating their marked potential as prognostic tools. In summary, this study presented a convincing methodology for the systematic development of multiparametric biomarker panels by machine learning. Yet, looking at the details of the initial biomarker selection, several obvious mistakes were made by paying too little attention to peculiarities of the analytical platforms and to previous experiences analyzing this data set, so there is certainly a lot of room for improvement regarding the diagnostic and prognostic performances.

In addition, the authors of this study also tested a combination of the three classifiers for its correlation with baseline and follow-up eGFR, but this approach did not significantly improve the correlation coefficients when compared to each of the three original biomarker panels. This may come as a surprise, even a disappointment, particularly considering the breakthroughs that could be achieved when conducting GWAS phenotypes defined by targeted metabolomics [81, 92]. Obviously, however, the fundamental belief of modern systems biology that the amassment of data from different omics disciplines would automatically generate such synergies (the more the merrier), is not necessarily true.

6. Summary and future perspectives

The present chapter attempted to summarize some of the latest breakthroughs in the identification and development of metabolic biomarkers for chronic renal failure. It is more than obvious that there is a huge unmet need for improved diagnostic and prognostic tools for this indication, which represents an immense—and continuously growing—burden for affected patients and public budgets alike. Also, the introduction and impressive clinical validation of more aggressive and personalized intervention strategies has further stressed the necessity for finding and implementing better markers for accurate staging of the disease, monitoring its progression or the effects of therapeutic regimens and, eventually, assessing each patient's individual prognosis to make early and informed decisions in disease management.

In the last decade, the entire armamentarium of bioanalytical platform technologies has been used in this quest. While genomic analyses identified certain risk factors and elucidated some new regulatory relationships, it was primarily proteomics and metabolomics, that is, the disciplines depicting functional endpoints rather than predispositions that reported findings with the potential for clinical application in the foreseeable future.

The statistical basis for these developments and, thus, their credibility has been strengthened substantially in the last few years when large population-based cohorts were analyzed in addition to the smaller, dedicated studies, in which clinical research was initially conducted. So, today, there are highly promising biomarker candidates to be developed as diagnostic tools that are not just backed by single observations but have been confirmed in independent cohorts, some even in comprehensive meta-analyses (e.g. SDMA), and many of them could be substantiated by research on relevant animal models and by a thorough elucidation of the underlying mechanisms, pathways, and networks.

Yet, so far, these data have often come from retrospective studies (at least, from retrospective data analyses), and (too) many of these studies have been based on eGFR-related inclusion and classification criteria (or rather fuzzy diagnostic parameters like micro-albuminuria, which is no longer considered a relevant clinical endpoint). Despite sophisticated statistical strategies and detailed additional phenotyping of the patients, the lack of large, prospective studies designed around hard clinical endpoints like mortality, initiation of RRT (or mGFR as a better measure of renal function, for that matter) still limits the dissemination and acceptance of these findings. The next couple of years, however, will witness the completion—or, at any rate, meaningful interim analyses—of presently ongoing studies that fulfill some of these essential criteria such as the PROVALID study initiated by the SysKid consortium [193], the German Kidney Disease (GCKD) Study [194], the UroSysteOmics study [61, 89, 91, 113, 183], the French Chronic Kidney Disease-Renal Epidemiology and Information Network (CKD-REIN) cohort study [195], the Proteomic prediction and Renin angiotensin aldosterone system Inhibition prevention Of early diabetic nephRopathy In TYpe 2 diabetic patients with normoalbuminuria (PRIORITY) trial [65], or the KoreaN cohort study for Outcome in patients With Chronic Kidney Disease (KNOW-CKD) [196], and these studies will be complemented and extended by both general and dedicated biobanking activities [197–200]. In the end, the data generated in these studies will hopefully facilitate a reasonable validation of some of the putative marker candidates presented in this chapter.

Still, the question remains, how close this will take the field to new, broadly available diagnostic tools in daily clinical practice? This issue will primarily depend on the technical feasibility and robustness in a routine setting such as clinical chemistry core facilities and the regulatory implications for the related products. For some of the most likely candidates to be successfully validated, these points can already be discussed in a fairly well-informed manner:

Starting with the proteomics output, the monoparametric protein markers, for example, KIM-1 or NGAL, can be quantified with reasonable accuracy and precision by standard immunoassays, and kits certified for *in vitro* diagnostics (IVD) use are commercially available, for example, from BioPorto Diagnostics (Hellerup, DK). The far more complex peptide and metabolite marker panels, however, have originally been discovered by MS (some also by NMR), and—as of today—there is hardly a plausible alternative platform that could replace mass spectrometric detection methods for these parameters—antibody-based detection is not suitable for small ubiquitous molecules like most of the metabolites discussed above, and the peptide panels would quickly exceed any reasonable limits for multiplexing immunoassays (at least on the currently established platforms). So, if MS is the method of choice for now (and for many technical reasons not to be discussed here, it will most likely stay this way for quite some time), what is the present status of clinical applications of MS? Of course, this strongly depends on three technicalities: (a) the kind of instrument used (triple quadrupole- or time-of-flight (ToF)-based platforms), (b) the separation step needed for a particular class of compounds, for example, none (flow injection analysis), capillary electrophoresis (CE), gas (GC), or liquid (LC) chromatography, and (c) the appropriate ionization technique, for example, electrospray (ESI) or photospray ionization (APPI), chemical ionization (CI), or matrix-assisted laser desorption ionization (MALDI). As for ToF-based systems, there is no routine application of a CE-ToF-MS platform in clinical routine today, and only a fairly recent adoption of a MALDI-ToF-MS instrument in bacteriology, the so-called MALDI Biotyper from Bruker (Billerica, MA, USA) [201]. In contrast, tandem mass spectrometry (MS/MS) using standard triple quadrupole (QqQ) instruments has been the gold standard in neonatal screening for two decades now [71, 72] with millions of newborns tested in an extremely sensitive and specific and, yet, highly cost-effective manner. Tandem MS is also an established component of state-of-the-art clinical chemistry labs in most industrialized countries by now and—notably—subject to stringent quality control [202, 203]. Routine applications of this platform range from therapeutic drug monitoring, most commonly for immunosuppressives [204], to assays for vitamin D and some if its metabolites [205], and from screening programs for drugs of abuse [206] to the worldwide anti-doping activities [207]. Moreover, the targeted portfolio is growing fast to also cover clinically relevant classes of compounds such as steroid hormones [208, 209], bile acids [210], catecholamines [211], and others.

As a matter of fact, the majority of the biomarker candidates presented in Section 4 (e.g. amino acids, biogenic amines, or acylcarnitines) are already amenable to standardized quantification by commercially available kit products, for example, as subsets of the AbsoluteIDQ™ portfolio from Biocrates (Innsbruck, AT). These kits are validated on most of the suitable mass spectrometers from the leading instrument vendors AB Sciex (Framingham, USA), Waters (Milford, USA), and Thermo Fisher (Waltham, USA), and the sample preparation procedures can be fully automated on robotic liquid handling systems, for example, from Hamilton (Bonaduz, CH) or Tecan (Männedorf, CH). Most important in this context, technically very similar kits have already been certified as *in vitro* diagnostics (IVD) according to the European directive 98/79/EC (IVDD), for example, the Stero*IDQ*™ from Biocrates. Of course, the new European regulation 2017/746 (IVDR), published on May 5, 2017, sets more challenging standards for such a certificate but there is no reason to believe that this will undermine the suitability of MS-based assays for routine diagnostics in principle. In conclusion, the technicalities of bringing a diagnostic metabolite panel into routine clinical practice seem quite straightforward, so it will primarily depend on the actual performance of these marker candidates in the ongoing validation studies if and when they could become part of the standard diagnostic repertoire and patients could eventually benefit from an improved disease management for CKD.

Acknowledgements

Parts of this work have been funded by the EuroTransBio project UroSysteOmics and have been previously published [82].

Conflict of interest

The authors are joint inventors of the patent family published as PCT/EP2009/003926, which is assigned to Biocrates Life Sciences AG (Innsbruck, Austria), their former employer.

Author details

Ulrika Lundin[1] and Klaus M. Weinberger[2,3,4]*

*Address all correspondence to: klaus.weinberger@ext.umit.at

1 Sandoz GmbH, Kundl, Austria

2 Research Group for Clinical Bioinformatics, Institute for Electrical and Biomedical Engineering (IEBE), University for Health Sciences, Medical Informatics and Technology (UMIT), Hall in Tirol, Austria

3 sAnalytiCo Ltd, Belfast, United Kingdom

4 Weinberger and Weinberger Life Sciences Consulting, Lappersdorf, Germany

References

[1] Rogers EM. New Product Adoption and Diffusion. Journal of Consumer Research. 1976;**2**(4):290

[2] Berson SA, Yalow RS. General principles of radioimmunoassay. Clinica Chimica Acta. 2006;**369**(2):125-143

[3] Köhler G, Milstein C. Continuous cultures of fused cells secreting antibody of predefined specificity. Nature. 1975;**256**(5517):495-497

[4] Southern EM. Detection of specific sequences among DNA fragments separated by gel electrophoresis. Journal of Molecular Biology. 1975

[5] Towbin H, Staehelin T, Gordon J. Electrophoretic transfer of proteins from polyacryl-amide gels to nitrocellulose sheets: Procedure and some applications. Proceedings of the National Academy of Sciences. 1979;**76**(9):4350-4354

[6] Mullis K, Faloona F, Scharf S, Saiki R, Horn G, Erlich H. Specific enzymatic amplification of DNA in vitro: The polymerase chain reaction. Cold Spring Harbor Symposia on Quantitative Biology. 1986;**51**(Pt 1):263-273

[7] Sanger F, Coulson AR. A rapid method for determining sequences in DNA by primed synthesis with DNA polymerase. Journal of Molecular Biology. 1975;**94**(3):441-448

[8] Aronson JK. Monitoring therapy. British Journal of Clinical Pharmacology. 2005;**60**(3): 229-230

[9] Barsoum RS. Chronic kidney disease in the developing world. The New England Journal of Medicine. 2006;**354**(10):997-999

[10] Zhang Q-L, Rothenbacher D. Prevalence of chronic kidney disease in population-based studies: Systematic review. BMC Public Health. 2008;**8**(1):117

[11] Fishbane S, Hazzan AD, Halinski C, Mathew AT. Challenges and opportunities in late-stage chronic kidney disease. Clinical Kidney Journal. 2015;**8**(1):54-60

[12] Eckardt K-U, Coresh J, Devuyst O, Johnson RJ, Köttgen A, Levey AS, et al. Evolving importance of kidney disease: From subspecialty to global health burden. Lancet. 2013; **382**(9887):158-169

[13] Zhao Y-Y. Metabolomics in chronic kidney disease. Clinica Chimica Acta. 2013;**422**:59-69

[14] Centers for Disease Control and Prevention (CDC). Prevalence of chronic kidney disease and associated risk factors—United States, 1999-2004. MMWR. Morbidity and Mortality Weekly Report. 2007;**56**(8):161-165

[15] Coresh J, Selvin E, Stevens LA, Manzi J, Kusek JW, Eggers P, et al. Prevalence of chronic kidney disease in the United States. JAMA. 2007;**298**(17):2038

[16] Park CW. Diabetic kidney disease: From epidemiology to clinical perspectives. Diabetes and Metabolism Journal. 2014;**38**(4):252-260

[17] Vegter S, Perna A, Postma MJ, Navis G, Remuzzi G, Ruggenenti P. Sodium intake, ACE inhibition, and progression to ESRD. Journal of the American Society of Nephrology. 2012;**23**(1):165-173

[18] Alani H. Cardiovascular co-morbidity in chronic kidney disease: Current knowledge and future research needs. World Journal of Nephrology. 2014;**3**(4):156

[19] Foley R, Parfrey P, Sarnak M. Clinical epidemiology of cardiovascular disease in chronic renal disease. American Journal of Kidney Diseases. 1998;**32**(5):S112-S119

[20] Parfrey PS, Foley RN. The clinical epidemiology of cardiac disease in chronic renal failure. Journal of the American Society of Nephrology. 1999;**10**(7):1606-1615

[21] Couser WG, Remuzzi G, Mendis S, Tonelli M. The contribution of chronic kidney disease to the global burden of major noncommunicable diseases. Kidney International. 2011;**80**(12):1258-1270

[22] Levey AS, Atkins R, Coresh J, Cohen EP, Collins AJ, Eckardt K-U, et al. Chronic kidney disease as a global public health problem: Approaches and initiatives—a position statement from Kidney Disease Improving Global Outcomes. Kidney International. 2007;**72**(3):247-259

[23] United States Renal Data System. Annual data report. 2013

[24] Grassmann A, Gioberge S, Moeller S, Brown G. ESRD patients in 2004: Global overview of patient numbers, treatment modalities and associated trends. Nephrology Dialysis Transplantation. 2005;**20**(12):2587-2593

[25] El Nahas AM, Bello AK. Chronic kidney disease: The global challenge. Lancet. 2005; 365(9456):331 340

[26] Cockcroft DW, Gault H. Prediction of creatinine clearance from serum creatinine. Nephron. 1976;**16**(1):31-41

[27] Huttunen N-P, Taalikka M, Metsola R. Sources of error in estimation of glomerular filtration rate from plasma creatinine concentration in children. Archives of Disease in Childhood. 1978;**53**(2):182-183

[28] Levey AS. A more accurate method to estimate glomerular filtration rate from serum creatinine: A new prediction equation. Annals of Internal Medicine. 1999;**130**(6):461

[29] Levey AS, Coresh J, Greene T, Stevens LA, Zhang Y, Hendriksen S, et al. Using standardized serum creatinine values in the modification of diet in renal disease study equation for estimating glomerular filtration rate. Annals of Internal Medicine. 2006;**145**(4):247

[30] Issa N, Meyer KH, Arrigain S, Choure G, Fatica RA, Nurko S, et al. Evaluation of creatinine-based estimates of glomerular filtration rate in a large Cohort of living kidney donors. Transplantation. 2008;**86**(2):223-230

[31] Murata K, Baumann NA, Saenger AK, Larson TS, Rule AD, Lieske JC. Relative performance of the MDRD and CKD-EPI equations for estimating glomerular filtration rate among patients with varied clinical presentations. Clinical Journal of the American Society of Nephrology. 2011;**6**(8):1963-1972

[32] Zhao W-Y, Zeng L, Zhu Y-H, Wang L-M, Zhou M-S, Han S, et al. A comparison of prediction equations for estimating glomerular filtration rate in Chinese potential living kidney donors. Clinical Transplantation. 2009;**23**(4):469-475

[33] Hauer HA, Bajema IM, Van Houwelingen HC, Ferrario F, Noël L-H, Waldherr R, et al. Determinants of outcome in ANCA-associated glomerulonephritis: A prospective clinico-histopathological analysis of 96 patients. Kidney International. 2002;**62**(5):1732-1742

[34] Levey AS, Inker LA, Coresh J. GFR estimation: From physiology to public health. American Journal of Kidney Diseases. 2014;**63**(5):820-834

[35] Tent H, Rook M, Stevens LA, van Son WJ, van Pelt LJ, Hofker HS, et al. Renal function equations before and after living kidney donation: A within-individual comparison of performance at different levels of renal function. Clinical Journal of the American Society of Nephrology. 2010;**5**(11):1960-1968

[36] Matas AJ, Smith JM, Skeans MA, Thompson B, Gustafson SK, Stewart DE, et al. OPTN/ SRTR 2013 Annual Data Report: Kidney. American Journal of Transplantation. 2015;**15**(S2): 1-34

[37] Mehrabi A, Fonouni H, Golriz M, Schmied B, Tahmasbirad M, Weitz J, et al. Lebendspende-Nierentransplantation. Der Chir. 2010;**81**(9):794-803

[38] Terasaki PI, Cecka JM, Gjertson DW, Takemoto S. High survival rates of kidney transplants from spousal and living unrelated donors. New England Journal of Medicine. 1995;**333**(6):333-336

[39] Hou FF, Xie D, Zhang X, Chen PY, Zhang WR, Liang M, et al. Renoprotection of Optimal Antiproteinuric Doses (ROAD) study: A randomized controlled study of benazepril and losartan in chronic renal insufficiency. Journal of the American Society of Nephrology. 2007;**18**(6):1889-1898

[40] Ruggenenti P, Perticucci E, Cravedi P, Gambara V, Costantini M, Sharma SK, et al. Role of remission clinics in the longitudinal treatment of CKD. Journal of the American Society of Nephrology. 2008;**19**(6):1213-1224

[41] Ruggenenti P, Schieppati A, Remuzzi G. Progression, remission, regression of chronic renal diseases. Lancet. 2001;**357**(9268):1601-1608

[42] Böger CA, Heid IM. Chronic kidney disease: Novel insights from genome-wide association studies. Kidney & Blood Pressure Research. 2011;**34**(4):225-234

[43] Böger CA, Sedor JR. GWAS of diabetic nephropathy: Is the GENIE out of the bottle? PLoS Genetics. 2012;**8**(9):e1002989

[44] Chambers JC, Zhang W, Lord GM, van der Harst P, Lawlor DA, Sehmi JS, et al. Genetic loci influencing kidney function and chronic kidney disease. Nature Genetics. 2010; **42**(5):373-375

[45] Köttgen A. Genome-wide association studies in nephrology research. American Journal of Kidney Diseases. 2010;**56**(4):743-758

[46] Li Y, Köttgen A. Genetic investigations of kidney disease: Core curriculum 2013. American Journal of Kidney Diseases. 2013;**61**(5):832-844

[47] Okada Y, Sim X, Go MJ, Wu J-Y, Gu D, Takeuchi F, et al. Meta-analysis identifies multiple loci associated with kidney function-related traits in east Asian populations. Nature Genetics. 2012;**44**(8):904-909

[48] Price PM, Hirschhorn K, Safirstein RL. Chronic kidney disease and GWAS: "The proper study of mankind is man". Cell Metabolism. 2010;**11**(6):451-452

[49] Suhre K, Shin S-Y, Petersen A-K, Mohney RP, Meredith D, Wägele B, et al. Human metabolic individuality in biomedical and pharmaceutical research. Nature. 2011; **477**(7362):54-60

[50] Wuttke M, Schaefer F, Wong CS, Köttgen A. Genome-wide association studies in nephrology: Using known associations for data checks. American Journal of Kidney Diseases. 2015;**65**(2):217-222

[51] Ju W, Eichinger F, Bitzer M, Oh J, McWeeney S, Berthier CC, et al. Renal gene and protein expression signatures for prediction of kidney disease progression. The American Journal of Pathology. 2009;**174**(6):2073-2085

[52] Ko GJ, Grigoryev DN, Linfert D, Jang HR, Watkins T, Cheadle C, et al. Transcriptional analysis of kidneys during repair from AKI reveals possible roles for NGAL and KIM-1 as biomarkers of AKI-to-CKD transition. American Journal of Physiology. Renal Physiology. 2010;**298**(6):F1472-F1483

[53] Szeto C-C, Ching-Ha KB, Ka-Bik L, Mac-Moune LF, Cheung-Lung CP, Gang W, et al. Micro-RNA expression in the urinary sediment of patients with chronic kidney diseases. Disease Markers. 2012;**33**(3):137-144

[54] Zaza G, Granata S, Rascio F, Pontrelli P, Dell'Oglio MP, Cox SN, et al. A specific immune transcriptomic profile discriminates chronic kidney disease patients in predialysis from hemodialyzed patients. BMC Medical Genomics. 2013;**6**(1):17

[55] Zawada AM, Rogacev KS, Müller S, Rotter B, Winter P, Fliser D, et al. Massive analysis of cDNA Ends (MACE) and miRNA expression profiling identifies proatherogenic pathways in chronic kidney disease. Epigenetics. 2014;**9**(1):161-172

[56] Konvalinka A. Urine proteomics for acute kidney injury prognosis: Another player and the long road ahead. Kidney International. 2014;**85**(4):735-738

[57] Lopez-Giacoman S. Biomarkers in chronic kidney disease, from kidney function to kidney damage. World Journal of Nephrology. 2015;**4**(1):57

[58] Filip S, Pontillo C, Peter Schanstra J, Vlahou A, Mischak H, Klein J. Urinary proteomics and molecular determinants of chronic kidney disease: Possible link to proteases. Expert Review of Proteomics. 2014;**11**(5):535-548

[59] Argilés À, Siwy J, Duranton F, Gayrard N, Dakna M, Lundin U, et al. CKD273, a new proteomics classifier assessing CKD and its prognosis. Rouet P, editor. PLoS One. 2013;**8**(5):e62837

[60] Critselis E, Lambers Heerspink H. Utility of the CKD273 peptide classifier in predicting chronic kidney disease progression. Nephrology, Dialysis, Transplantation. 2016;**31**(2):249-254

[61] Gu Y-M, Thijs L, Liu Y-P, Zhang Z, Jacobs L, Koeck T, et al. The urinary proteome as correlate and predictor of renal function in a population study. Nephrology, Dialysis, Transplantation. 2014;**29**(12):2260-2268

[62] Schanstra JP, Mischak H. Proteomic urinary biomarker approach in renal disease: From discovery to implementation. Pediatric Nephrology. 2015;**30**(5):713-725

[63] Siwy J, Schanstra JP, Argiles A, Bakker SJL, Beige J, Boucek P, et al. Multicentre prospective validation of a urinary peptidome-based classifier for the diagnosis of type 2 diabetic nephropathy. Nephrology, Dialysis, Transplantation. 2014;**29**(8):1563-1570

[64] Altmaier E, Ramsay SL, Graber A, Mewes H-W, Weinberger KM, Suhre K. Bioinformatics analysis of targeted metabolomics—Uncovering old and new tales of diabetic mice under medication. Endocrinology. 2008;**149**(7):3478-3489

[65] Floegel A, Stefan N, Yu Z, Muhlenbruch K, Drogan D, Joost H-G, et al. Identification of serum metabolites associated with risk of type 2 diabetes using a targeted metabolomic approach. Diabetes. 2013;**62**(2):639-648

[66] Wang TJ, Larson MG, Vasan RS, Cheng S, Rhee EP, McCabe E, et al. Metabolite profiles and the risk of developing diabetes. Nature Medicine. 2011;**17**(4):448-453

[67] Wang-Sattler R, Yu Z, Herder C, Messias AC, Floegel A, He Y, et al. Novel biomarkers for pre-diabetes identified by metabolomics. Molecular Systems Biology. 2012;**8**:615

[68] Weinberger KM. Metabolomics in diagnosing metabolic diseases. Therapeutische Umschau. Revue Thérapeutique. 2008;**65**(9):487-491

[69] Würtz P, Soininen P, Kangas AJ, Rönnemaa T, Lehtimäki T, Kähönen M, et al. Branched-chain and aromatic amino acids are predictors of insulin resistance in young adults. Diabetes Care. 2013;**36**(3):648-655

[70] Chace DH. Use of tandem mass spectrometry for multianalyte screening of dried blood specimens from newborns. Clinical Chemistry. 2003;**49**(11):1797-1817

[71] Röschinger W, Olgemöller B, Fingerhut R, Liebl B, Roscher AA. Advances in analytical mass spectrometry to improve screening for inherited metabolic diseases. European Journal of Pediatrics. 2003;**162**:S67-S76

[72] Weinberger KM, Graber A, Katzenberger J. Targeted metabolomics. Biospektrum. 2006;**12**(2):231-232

[73] Weinberger KM, Graber A. Using comprehensive metabolomics to identify novel biomarkers. Screening Trends in Drug Discovery. 2005;**6**:42-45

[74] Fassett RG, Venuthurupalli SK, Gobe GC, Coombes JS, Cooper MA, Hoy WE. Biomarkers in chronic kidney disease: A review. Kidney International. 2011;**80**(8):806-821

[75] McMahon GM, Waikar SS. Biomarkers in nephrology: Core curriculum 2013. American Journal of Kidney Diseases. 2013;**62**(1):165-178

[76] Hocher B, Adamski J. Metabolomics for clinical use and research in chronic kidney disease. Nature Reviews Nephrology. 2017;**13**(5):269-284

[77] Breit M, Baumgartner C, Weinberger KM. Data handling and analysis in metabolomics. In: Khanmohammadi M, editor. Current Applications of Chemometrics. New York: Nova Science Publishers; 2015. pp. 181-203

[78] Enot DP, Haas B, Weinberger KM. Bioinformatics for mass spectrometry-based metabolomics. Methods in Molecular Biology (Clifton, NJ). 2011. pp. 351-375

[79] Gieger C, Geistlinger L, Altmaier E, Hrabé de Angelis M, Kronenberg F, Meitinger T, et al. Genetics meets metabolomics: A genome-wide association study of metabolite profiles in human serum. Gibson G, editor. PLoS Genet. 2008;**4**(11):e1000282

[80] Breit M, Weinberger KM. Metabolic biomarkers for chronic kidney disease. Archives of Biochemistry and Biophysics. 2016;**589**:62-80

[81] Bode-Böger SM, Scalera F, Kielstein JT, Martens-Lobenhoffer J, Breithardt G, Fobker M, et al. Symmetrical dimethylarginine: A new combined parameter for renal function and extent of coronary artery disease. Journal of the American Society of Nephrology. 2006;**17**(4):1128-1134

[82] Fleck C, Schweitzer F, Karge E, Busch M, Stein G. Serum concentrations of asymmetric (ADMA) and symmetric (SDMA) dimethylarginine in patients with chronic kidney diseases. Clinica Chimica Acta. 2003;**336**(1-2):1-12

[83] Leone A, Moncada S, Vallance P, Calver A, Collier J. Accumulation of an endogenous inhibitor of nitric oxide synthesis in chronic renal failure. Lancet. 1992;**339**(8793):572-575

[84] Krause CD, Yang Z-H, Kim Y-S, Lee J-H, Cook JR, Pestka S. Protein arginine methyltransferases: Evolution and assessment of their pharmacological and therapeutic potential. Pharmacology and Therapeutics. 2007;**113**(1):50-87

[85] Böger RH, Maas R, Schulze F, Schwedhelm E. Elevated levels of asymmetric dimethylarginine (ADMA) as a marker of cardiovascular disease and mortality. Clinical Chemistry and Laboratory Medicine. 2005;**43**(10):1124-1129

[86] Dimitroulas T, Sandoo A, Kitas GD. Asymmetric dimethylarginine as a surrogate marker of endothelial dysfunction and cardiovascular risk in patients with systemic rheumatic diseases. International Journal of Molecular Sciences. 2012;**13**(12):12315-12335

[87] Lundin U, Modre-Osprian R, Weinberger KM. Targeted metabolomics for clinical biomarker discovery in multifactorial diseases. In: Ikehara K, editor. Genetic Disorders. Rijeka: InTech; 2011. pp. 81-98

[88] Robinson S, Pool R, Giffin R. Emerging Safety Science. Washington: The National Academies Press; 2008

[89] Duranton F, Lundin U, Gayrard N, Mischak H, Aparicio M, Mourad G, et al. Plasma and urinary amino acid metabolomic profiling in patients with different levels of kidney function. Clinical Journal of the American Society of Nephrology. 2014;**9**(1):37-45

[90] Illig T, Gieger C, Zhai G, Römisch-Margl W, Wang-Sattler R, Prehn C, et al. A genome-wide perspective of genetic variation in human metabolism. Nature Genetics. 2010; **42**(2):137-141

[91] Weikard R, Altmaier E, Suhre K, Weinberger KM, Hammon HM, Albrecht E, et al. Metabolomic profiles indicate distinct physiological pathways affected by two loci with major divergent effect on Bos taurus growth and lipid deposition. Physiological Genomics. 2010;**42A**(2):79-88

[92] Kielstein JT, Salpeter SR, Bode-Boeger SM, Cooke JP, Fliser D. Symmetric dimethylarginine (SDMA) as endogenous marker of renal function—A meta-analysis. Nephrology, Dialysis, Transplantation. 2006;**21**(9):2446-2451

[93] Fleck C, Janz A, Schweitzer F, Karge E, Schwertfeger M, Stein G. Serum concentrations of asymmetric (ADMA) and symmetric (SDMA) dimethylarginine in renal failure patients. Kidney International. Supplement. 2001;**78**:S14-S18

[94] Berger M, Gray JA, Roth BL. The expanded biology of serotonin. Annual Review of Medicine. 2009;**60**(1):355-366

[95] Hardeland R, Pandi-Perumal SR, Cardinali DP. Melatonin. The international Journal of Biochemistry & Cell Biology. 2006;**38**(3):313-316

[96] Harden JL, Egilmez NK. Indoleamine 2,3-dioxygenase and dendritic cell tolerogenicity. Immunological Investigations. 2012;**41**(6-7):738-764

[97] Johnson TS, Munn DH. Host indoleamine 2,3-dioxygenase: Contribution to systemic acquired tumor tolerance. Immunological Investigations. 2012;**41**(6-7):765-797

[98] Munn DH, Mellor AL. Indoleamine 2,3 dioxygenase and metabolic control of immune responses. Trends in Immunology. 2013;**34**(3):137-143

[99] Kotake Y, Masayama T. Stadien über den intermediären Stoffwechsel des Tryptophans XVIII. Über den Mechanismus der Kynurenin-bildung aus Tryptophan. Zeitschrift für Physiol Chemie. 1936

[100] Takikawa O. Biochemical and medical aspects of the indoleamine 2,3-dioxygenase-initiated l-tryptophan metabolism. Biochemical and Biophysical Research Communications. 2005;**338**(1):12-19

[101] Ozaki M. Metabolism of monoamines in spontaneously hypertensive rats. Japanese Journal of Pharmacology. 1966;**16**(3):257-263

[102] Egashira Y, Nagaki S, Sanada H. Tryptophan-Niacin metabolism in rat with puromycin aminonucleoside-induced nephrosis. International Journal for Vitamin and Nutrition Research. 2006;**76**(1):28-33

[103] Saito K, Fujigaki S, Heyes MP, Shibata K, Takemura M, Fujii H, et al. Mechanism of increases in L-kynurenine and quinolinic acid in renal insufficiency. American Journal of Physiology—Renal Physiology. 2000;**279**(3):F565-F572

[104] Zhao Y-Y, Cheng X-L, Wei F, Xiao X-Y, Sun W-J, Zhang Y, et al. Serum metabonomics study of adenine-induced chronic renal failure in rats by ultra performance liquid chromatography coupled with quadrupole time-of-flight mass spectrometry. Biomarkers. 2012;**17**(1):48-55

[105] Zhao Y-Y, Liu J, Cheng X-L, Bai X, Lin R-C. Urinary metabonomics study on biochemical changes in an experimental model of chronic renal failure by adenine based on UPLC Q-TOF/MS. Clinica Chimica Acta. 2012;**413**(5-6):642-649

[106] Altmaier E, Kastenmüller G, Römisch-Margl W, Thorand B, Weinberger KM, Illig T, et al. Questionnaire-based self-reported nutrition habits associate with serum metabolism as revealed by quantitative targeted metabolomics. European Journal of Epidemiology. 2011;**26**(2):145-156

[107] Breier M, Wahl S, Prehn C, Fugmann M, Ferrari U, Weise M, et al. Targeted metabolomics identifies reliable and stable metabolites in human serum and plasma samples. PLoS One. 2014;**9**(2):e89728

[108] Jaremek M, Yu Z, Mangino M, Mittelstrass K, Prehn C, Singmann P, et al. Alcohol-induced metabolomic differences in humans. Translational Psychiatry. 2013;**3**(7):e276

[109] Netzer M, Kugler KG, Müller LAJ, Weinberger KM, Graber A, Baumgartner C, et al. A network-based feature selection approach to identify metabolic signatures in disease. Journal of Theoretical Biology. 2012;**310**:216-222

[110] Pichler Hefti J, Sonntag D, Hefti U, Risch L, Schoch OD, Turk AJ, et al. Oxidative stress in hypobaric hypoxia and influence on vessel-tone modifying mediators. High Altitude Medicine & Biology. 2013;**14**(3):273-279

[111] Wang-Sattler R, Yu Y, Mittelstrass K, Lattka E, Altmaier E, Gieger C, et al. Metabolic profiling reveals distinct variations linked to nicotine consumption in humans—First results from the KORA study. PLoS One. 2008;**3**(12):e3863

[112] Lundin U. Biomarker Discovery in Diabetic Nephropathy by Targeted Metabolomics. Linköping, Sweden: Linköping University; 2008

[113] Lundin U, Weinberger KM. New biomarkers for assessing kidney diseases. WO/2010/139341, 2010

[114] Goek O-N, Prehn C, Sekula P, Römisch-Margl W, Döring A, Gieger C, et al. Metabolites associate with kidney function decline and incident chronic kidney disease in the general population. Nephrology, Dialysis, Transplantation. 2013;**28**(8):2131-2138

[115] Goek O-N, Döring A, Gieger C, Heier M, Koenig W, Prehn C, et al. Serum metabolite concentrations and decreased GFR in the general population. American Journal of Kidney Diseases. 2012;**60**(2):197-206

[116] McMenamy RH, Oncley JL. The specific binding of L-tryptophan to serum albumin. The Journal of Biological Chemistry. 1958;**233**(6):1436-1447

[117] Sasaki E, Ohta Y, Shinohara R, Ishiguro I. Contribution of serum albumin to the transport of orally administered L-tryptophan into liver of rats with L-tryptophan depletion. Amino Acids. 1999;**16**(1):29-39

[118] Wurtman RJ. Tryptophan. In: Adelman G, Smith BH, editors. Encyclopedia of Neuroscience. Amsterdam: Elsevier; 2004

[119] Barreto FC, Barreto D V., Liabeuf S, Meert N, Glorieux G, Temmar M, et al. Serum indoxyl sulfate is associated with vascular disease and mortality in chronic kidney disease patients. Clinical Journal of the American Society of Nephrology. 2009;**4**(10):1551-1558

[120] Niwa T. Indoxyl sulfate is a nephro-vascular toxin. Journal of Renal Nutrition. 2010;**20**(5):S2-S6

[121] Yoshikawa D, Ishii H, Suzuki S, Takeshita K, Kumagai S, Hayashi M, et al. Plasma indoxyl sulfate and estimated glomerular filtration rate. Circulation Journal. 2014;**78**(10): 2477-2482

[122] Ramezani A, Raj DS. The gut microbiome, kidney disease, and targeted interventions. Journal of the American Society of Nephrology. 2014;**25**(4):657-670

[123] Saito A, Takagi T, Chung TG, Ohta K. Serum levels of polyamines in patients with chronic renal failure. Kidney International. Supplement. 1983;**16**:S234-S237

[124] Swendseid ME, Panaqua M, Kopple JD. Polyamine concentrations in red cells and urine of patients with chronic renal failure. Life Sciences. 1980;**26**(7):533-539

[125] Durante W, Johnson FK, Johnson RA. Arginase: A critical regulator of nitric oxide synthesis and vascular function. Clinical and Experimental Pharmacology and Physiology. 2007;**34**(9):906-911

[126] Baylis C. Nitric oxide deficiency in chronic kidney disease. American Journal of Physiology. Renal Physiology. 2008;**294**(1):F1-F9

[127] Hirayama A, Nakashima E, Sugimoto M, Akiyama S, Sato W, Maruyama S, et al. Metabolic profiling reveals new serum biomarkers for differentiating diabetic nephropathy. Analytical and Bioanalytical Chemistry. 2012;**404**(10):3101-3109

[128] Shah VO, Townsend RR, Feldman HI, Pappan KL, Kensicki E, Vander Jagt DL. Plasma metabolomic profiles in different stages of CKD. Clinical Journal of the American Society of Nephrology. 2013;**8**(3):363-370

[129] Baud L, Ardaillou R. Reactive oxygen species: Production and role in the kidney. American Journal of Physiology. 1986;**251**(5 Pt 2):F765-F776

[130] Gugliucci A, Menini T. The axis AGE-RAGE-soluble RAGE and oxidative stress in chronic kidney disease. In: Advances in Experimental Medicine and Biology. 2014. pp. 191-208

[131] Hagmann H, Brinkkoetter PT. ROS and oxidative stress in CKD patients: Is it the mitochondria that keeps CKD patients in bed? Nephrology Dialysis Transplantation. 2015;**30**(6):867-868

[132] Sharma K. Obesity, oxidative stress, and fibrosis in chronic kidney disease. Kidney International Supplements. 2014;**4**(1):113-117

[133] Sung C-C, Hsu Y-C, Chen C-C, Lin Y-F, Wu C-C. Oxidative stress and nucleic acid oxidation in patients with chronic kidney disease. Oxidative Medicine and Cellular Longevity. 2013;**2013**:301982

[134] Bartosz G. Peroxynitrite: Mediator of the toxic action of nitric oxide. Acta Biochimica Polonica. 1996;**43**(4):645-659

[135] Imlay J, Linn S. DNA damage and oxygen radical toxicity. Science. 1988;**240**(4857): 1302-1309

[136] Porter NA, Caldwell SE, Mills KA. Mechanisms of free radical oxidation of unsaturated lipids. Lipids. 1995;**30**(4):277-290

[137] Souza JM, Peluffo G, Radi R. Protein tyrosine nitration—Functional alteration or just a biomarker? Free Radical Biology and Medicine. 2008;**45**(4):357-366

[138] Chao M-R, Hsu Y-W, Liu H-H, Lin J-H, Hu C W. Simultaneous detection of 3-nitrotyrosine and 3-nitro-4-hydroxyphenylacetic acid in human urine by online SPE LC-MS/MS and their association with oxidative and methylated DNA lesions. Chemical Research in Toxicology. 2015;**28**(5):997-1006

[139] Tsikas D, Mitschke A, Gutzki F-M. Measurement of 3-nitro-tyrosine in human plasma and urine by gas chromatography-tandem mass spectrometry. Methods in Molecular Biology (Clifton, NJ). 2012:255-270

[140] Jäger W, Gruber A, Giessrigl B, Krupitza G, Szekeres T, Sonntag D. Metabolomic analysis of resveratrol-induced effects in the human breast cancer cell lines MCF-7 and MDA-MB-231. OMICS. 2011;**15**(1-2):9-14

[141] Krug AK, Gutbier S, Zhao L, Pöltl D, Kullmann C, Ivanova V, et al. Transcriptional and metabolic adaptation of human neurons to the mitochondrial toxicant MPP+. Cell Death and Disease. 2014;**5**(5):e1222

[142] Vogt W. Oxidation of methionyl residues in proteins: Tools, targets, and reversal. Free Radical Biology and Medicine. 1995;**18**(1):93-105

[143] Kopple JD. Phenylalanine and tyrosine metabolism in chronic kidney failure. Journal of Nutrition. 2007;**137**(6 Suppl 1):1586S-1590S; discussion 1597S-1598S

[144] Sonntag D, Koal T, Ramsay SL, Dammeier S, Weinberger KM, Unterwurzacher I. Inflammation and oxidative stress level assay. WO/2008/145384, 2008

[145] Weinberger KM, Graber A, Ramsay SL. Biomarker and method for determining an oxidative stress level. WO/2008/145385, 2008

[146] Werner ER, Blau N, Thöny B. Tetrahydrobiopterin: Biochemistry and pathophysiology. The Biochemical Journal. 2011;**438**(3):397-414

[147] Bremer J. Carnitine-metabolism and functions. Physiological Reviews. 1983;**63**(4): 1420-1480

[148] Bremer J. The role of carnitine in intracellular metabolism. Journal of Clinical Chemistry and Clinical Biochemistry. 1990;**28**(5):297-301

[149] Mitchell ME. Carnitine metabolism in human subjects. I. Normal metabolism. American Journal of Clinical Nutrition. 1978;**31**(2):293-306

[150] Ramsay SL, Stöggl W, Weinberger KM, Graber A, Guggenbichler W. Apparatus and method for analyzing a metabolite profile. WO/2007/003343, 2007

[151] Ramsay SL, Guggenbichler W, Weinberger KM, Graber A, Stöggl W. Device for quantitative analysis of a drug or metabolite profile. WO/2007/003344, 2007

[152] Hedlund GL, Longo N, Pasquali M. Glutaric acidemia type 1. American Journal of Medical Genetics Part C: Seminars in Medical Genetics. 2006;**142C**(2):86-94

[153] Kölker S, Christensen E, Leonard J V., Greenberg CR, Boneh A, Burlina AB, et al. Diagnosis and management of glutaric aciduria type I-revised recommendations. Journal of Inherited Metabolic Disease. 2011;**34**(3):677-694

[154] Choi J-Y, Yoon YJ, Choi H-J, Park S-H, Kim C-D, Kim I-S, et al. Dialysis modality-dependent changes in serum metabolites: Accumulation of inosine and hypoxanthine in patients on haemodialysis. Nephrology Dialysis Transplantation. 2011;**26**(4):1304-1313

[155] Duan H, Guan N, Wu Y, Zhang J, Ding J, Shao B. Identification of biomarkers for melamine-induced nephrolithiasis in young children based on ultra high performance liquid chromatography coupled to time-of-flight mass spectrometry (U-HPLC–Q-TOF/MS). Journal of Chromatography, B: Analytical Technologies in the Biomedical and Life Sciences. 2011;**879**(30):3544-3550

[156] Hayashi, Hiroyuki S, Takako H, Makoto S, Satsuki I, Tomoyoshi S, et al. Use of serum and urine metabolome analysis for the detection of metabolic changes in patients with stage 1-2 chronic kidney disease. Nephro-Urology Monthly. 2011

[157] Jia L, Chen J, Yin P, Lu X, Xu G. Serum metabonomics study of chronic renal failure by ultra performance liquid chromatography coupled with Q-TOF mass spectrometry. Metabolomics. 2008;**4**(2):183-189

[158] Ma C, Bi K, Su D, Ji W, Zhang M, Fan X, et al. Serum and kidney metabolic changes of rat nephrotoxicity induced by Morning Glory Seed. Food and Chemical Toxicology. 2010;**48**(10):2988-2993

[159] Mishima E, Inoue C, Saigusa D, Inoue R, Ito K, Suzuki Y, et al. Conformational change in transfer RNA is an early indicator of acute cellular damage. Journal of the American Society of Nephrology. 2014;**25**(10):2316-2326

[160] Psihogios NG, Kalaitzidis RG, Dimou S, Seferiadis KI, Siamopoulos KC, Bairaktari ET. Evaluation of tubulointerstitial lesions' severity in patients with glomerulonephritides: An NMR-based metabonomic study. Journal of Proteome Research. 2007;**6**(9):3760-3770

[161] Qi S, Ouyang X, Wang L, Peng W, Wen J, Dai Y. A pilot metabolic profiling study in serum of patients with chronic kidney disease based on 1 H-NMR-spectroscopy. Clinical and Translational Science. 2012;**5**(5):379-385

[162] Rhee EP, Souza A, Farrell L, Pollak MR, Lewis GD, Steele DJR, et al. Metabolite profiling identifies markers of uremia. Journal of the American Society of Nephrology. 2010;**21**(6):1041-1051

[163] Sato E, Kohno M, Yamamoto M, Fujisawa T, Fujiwara K, Tanaka N. Metabolomic analysis of human plasma from haemodialysis patients. European Journal of Clinical Investigation. 2011;**41**(3):241-255

[164] Sui W, Li L, Che W, Zuo G, Chen J, Li W, et al. A proton nuclear magnetic resonance-based metabonomics study of metabolic profiling in immunoglobulin a nephropathy. Clinics. 2012;**67**(4):363-373

[165] Wikoff WR, Nagle MA, Kouznetsova VL, Tsigelny IF, Nigam SK. Untargeted metabolomics identifies enterobiome metabolites and putative uremic toxins as substrates of organic anion transporter 1 (Oat1) Journal of Proteome Research. 2011;**10**(6):2042-2051

[166] Zhang J, Yan L, Chen W, Lin L, Song X, Yan X, et al. Metabonomics research of diabetic nephropathy and type 2 diabetes mellitus based on UPLC–oaTOF-MS system. Analytica Chimica Acta. 2009;**650**(1):16-22

[167] Zhao Y-Y, Lin R-C. Metabolomics in nephrotoxicity. In: Advances in Clinical Chemistry. 2014. pp. 69-89

[168] Zhao Y-Y, Cheng X-L, Wei F, Bai X, Lin R-C. Application of faecal metabonomics on an experimental model of tubulointerstitial fibrosis by ultra performance liquid chromatography/high-sensitivity mass spectrometry with MS E data collection technique. Biomarkers. 2012;**17**(8):721-729

[169] Zhao Y-Y, Shen X, Cheng X-L, Wei F, Bai X, Lin R-C. Urinary metabonomics study on the protective effects of ergosta-4,6,8(14),22-tetraen-3-one on chronic renal failure in rats using UPLC Q-TOF/MS and a novel MSE data collection technique. Process Biochemistry. 2012;**47**(12):1980-1987

[170] Zhao Y-Y, Zhang L, Long F-Y, Cheng X-L, Bai X, Wei F, et al. UPLC-Q-TOF/HSMS/MSE-based metabonomics for adenine-induced changes in metabolic profiles of rat faeces and intervention effects of ergosta-4,6,8(14),22-tetraen-3-one. Chemico-Biological Interactions. 2013;**201**(1-3):31-38

[171] Zhao Y-Y, Li H-T, Feng Y-L, Bai X, Lin R-C. Urinary metabonomic study of the surface layer of Poria cocos as an effective treatment for chronic renal injury in rats. Journal of Ethnopharmacology. 2013;**148**(2):403-410

[172] Zhao Y-Y, Lei P, Chen D-Q, Feng Y-L, Bai X. Renal metabolic profiling of early renal injury and renoprotective effects of Poria cocos epidermis using UPLC Q-TOF/HSMS/MSE. Journal of Pharmaceutical and Biomedical Analysis. 2013;**81-82**:202-209

[173] Huang X, Sjögren P, Ärnlöv J, Cederholm T, Lind L, Stenvinkel P, et al. Serum fatty acid patterns, insulin sensitivity and the metabolic syndrome in individuals with chronic kidney disease. Journal of Internal Medicine. 2014;**275**(1):71-83

[174] Suhre K, Meisinger C, Döring A, Altmaier E, Belcredi P, Gieger C, et al. Metabolic footprint of diabetes: A multiplatform metabolomics study in an epidemiological setting. Breant B, editor. PLoS One. 2010;**5**(11):e13953

[175] Altmaier E, Kastenmüller G, Römisch-Margl W, Thorand B, Weinberger KM, Adamski J, et al. Variation in the human lipidome associated with coffee consumption as revealed by quantitative targeted metabolomics. Molecular Nutrition & Food Research. 2009;**53**(11):1357-1365

[176] Quach ND, Arnold RD, Cummings BS. Secretory phospholipase A2 enzymes as pharmacological targets for treatment of disease. Biochemical Pharmacology. 2014;**90**(4): 338-348

[177] Unterwurzacher I, Koal T, Bonn GK, Weinberger KM, Ramsay SL. Rapid sample preparation and simultaneous quantitation of prostaglandins and lipoxygenase derived fatty acid metabolites by liquid chromatography-mass spectrometry from small sample volumes. Clinical Chemistry and Laboratory Medicine. 2008;**46**(11):1589-1597

[178] Weinberger KM, Breit M. Targeted metabolomics: The next generation of clinical chemistry!? In: Wang X, editor. Application of Clinical Bioinformatics. Dordrecht: Springer; 2016. pp. 173-209

[179] Baumgartner C. A clinical metabolomics strategy to discover new biomarkers in complex disease: An overview. Biomedizinische Technik. 2013

[180] Baumgartner C, Graber A. Data mining and knowledge discovery in metabolomics. In: Masseglia F, Poncelet P, Teisseire M, editors. Successes and New Directions in Data Mining. London: Information Science Reference; 2008. pp. 141-166

[181] Baumgartner C, Osl M, Netzer M, Baumgartner D. Bioinformatic-driven search for metabolic biomarkers in disease. Journal of Clinical Bioinformatics. 2011;**1**(1):2

[182] Breit M, Baumgartner C, Netzer M, Weinberger KM. Clinical bioinformatics for biomarker discovery in targeted metabolomics. In: Wang X, editor. Application of Clinical Bioinformatics. Dordrecht: Springer; 2016. pp. 211-238

[183] Nkuipou-Kenfack E, Duranton F, Gayrard N, Argilés À, Lundin U, Weinberger KM, et al. Assessment of metabolomic and proteomic biomarkers in detection and prognosis of progression of renal function in chronic kidney disease. Philippe Rouet PhD, editor. PLoS One. 2014;**9**(5):e96955

[184] Pena MJ, Lambers Heerspink HJ, Hellemons ME, Friedrich T, Dallmann G, Lajer M, et al. Urine and plasma metabolites predict the development of diabetic nephropathy in individuals with Type 2 diabetes mellitus. Diabetic Medicine. 2014;31(9):1138-1147

[185] Turing AM. Computing machinery and intelligence. Mind. 1950

[186] Bressmann T. Self-inflicted cosmetic tongue split: A case report. Journal Canadian Dental Association. 2004;70(3):156-157

[187] Samuel AL. Some studies in machine learning using the game of checkers. IBM Journal of Research and Development. 1959;3(3):210-229

[188] Solomonoff RJ. A formal theory of inductive inference. Part I. Information and Control. 1964;7(1):1-22

[189] Alpaydin E. Introduction to machine learning. Journal of Chemical Information and Modeling. 2013

[190] Domingos P. A few useful things to know about machine learning. Communications of the ACM. 2012;55(10):78

[191] Sebag M. A tour of machine learning: An AI perspective. AI Communications. 2014

[192] Boser BE, Guyon IM, Vapnik VN. A training algorithm for optimal margin classifiers. In: Proceedings of the Fifth Annual Workshop on Computational Learning Theory—COLT '92. New York, USA: ACM Press; 1992. pp. 144-152

[193] Eder S, Leierer J, Kerschbaum J, Rosivall L, Wiecek A, de Zeeuw D, et al. A prospective cohort study in patients with type 2 diabetes mellitus for validation of biomarkers (PROVALID)—Study design and baseline characteristics. Kidney & Blood Pressure Research. 2018;43(1):181-190

[194] Eckardt K-U, Barthlein B, Baid-Agrawal S, Beck A, Busch M, Eitner F, et al. The German Chronic Kidney Disease (GCKD) study: Design and methods. Nephrology Dialysis Transplantation. 2012;27(4):1454-1460

[195] Stengel B, Combe C, Jacquelinet C, Briancon S, Fouque D, Laville M, et al. The French chronic kidney disease-renal epidemiology and information network (CKD-REIN) cohort study. Nephrology Dialysis Transplantation. 2014;29(8):1500-1507

[196] Oh K-H, Park SK, Park HC, Chin HJ, Chae DW, Choi KH, et al. KNOW-CKD (KoreaN cohort study for Outcome in patients With Chronic Kidney Disease): Design and methods. BMC Nephrology. 2014;15(1):80

[197] Harris JR, Burton P, Knoppers BM, Lindpaintner K, Bledsoe M, Brookes AJ, et al. Toward a roadmap in global biobanking for health. European Journal of Human Genetics. 2012;20(11):1105-1111

[198] Navis GJ, Blankestijn PJ, Deegens J, De Fijter JW, Homan van der Heide JJ, Rabelink T, et al. The biobank of nephrological diseases in the Netherlands cohort: The String

of Pearls Initiative collaboration on chronic kidney disease in the university medical centers in the Netherlands. Nephrology Dialysis Transplantation. 2014;**29**(6):1145-1150

[199] van Ommen G-JB, Törnwall O, Bréchot C, Dagher G, Galli J, Hveem K, et al. BBMRI-ERIC as a resource for pharmaceutical and life science industries: The development of biobank-based Expert Centres. European Journal of Human Genetics. 2015;**23**(7):893-900

[200] Yuille M, van Ommen G-J, Brechot C, Cambon-Thomsen A, Dagher G, Landegren U, et al. Biobanking for Europe. Briefings in Bioinformatics. 2007;**9**(1):14-24

[201] Kaleta EJ, Clark AE, Cherkaoui A, Wysocki VH, Ingram EL, Schrenzel J, et al. Comparative analysis of PCR-electrospray ionization/mass spectrometry (MS) and MALDI-TOF/MS for the identification of bacteria and yeast from positive blood culture bottles. Clinical Chemistry. 2011;**57**(7):1057-1067

[202] Vogeser M, Seger C. A decade of HPLC–MS/MS in the routine clinical laboratory—Goals for further developments. Clinical Biochemistry. 2008;**41**(9):649-662

[203] Vogeser M, Seger C. Quality management in clinical application of mass spectrometry measurement systems. Clinical Biochemistry. 2016;**49**(13-14):947-954

[204] Seger C, Tentschert K, Stöggl W, Griesmacher A, Ramsay SL. A rapid HPLC-MS/MS method for the simultaneous quantification of cyclosporine A, tacrolimus, sirolimus and everolimus in human blood samples. Nature Protocols. 2009;**4**(4):526-534

[205] van den Ouweland JMW, Vogeser M, Bächer S. Vitamin D and metabolites measurement by tandem mass spectrometry. Reviews in Endocrine & Metabolic Disorders. 2013;**14**(2):159-184

[206] Lee Y-W. Simultaneous screening of 177 drugs of abuse in urine using ultra-performance liquid chromatography with tandem mass spectrometry in drug-intoxicated patients. Clinical Psychopharmacology and Neuroscience. 2013;**11**(3):158-164

[207] Thevis M, Thomas A, Schänzer W. Targeting prohibited substances in doping control blood samples by means of chromatographic–mass spectrometric methods. Analytical and Bioanalytical Chemistry. 2013;**405**(30):9655-9667

[208] Ackermans MT, Endert E. LC–MS/MS in endocrinology: What is the profit of the last 5 years? Bioanalysis. 2014;**6**(1):43-57

[209] Koal T, Schmiederer D, Pham-Tuan H, Röhring C, Rauh M. Standardized LC–MS/MS based steroid hormone profile-analysis. The Journal of Steroid Biochemistry and Molecular Biology. 2012;**129**(3-5):129-138

[210] Griffiths WJ, Sjovall J. Bile acids: Analysis in biological fluids and tissues. Journal of Lipid Research. 2010;**51**(1):23-41

[211] Bicker J, Fortuna A, Alves G, Falcão A. Liquid chromatographic methods for the quantification of catecholamines and their metabolites in several biological samples—A review. Analytica Chimica Acta. 2013;**768**:12-34

7

Alport Syndrome

Marina Aksenova and Lev Shagam

Abstract

Alport syndrome is a multisystem disorder including progressive renal disease, sensorineural deafness, and eye abnormalities. The high risk of cardiovascular pathology in patients with Alport syndrome was also described recently. The syndrome is caused by mutations in *COL4A3*, *COL4A4*, and *COL4A5* genes, which lead to defects in glomerular filtration barrier and other basement membrane. The diagnosis of Alport syndrome should be suspected in patients with glomerular hematuria and with family history of renal failure. The severity of the individual symptoms and renal prognosis are variable and depend on gene mutation type. The current standard of treatment is the use of angiotensin-converting enzyme inhibitors, which delay the progression of renal failure in Alport syndrome. The recent knowledge in pathogenesis of disease opens new therapeutic perspectives.

Keywords: Alport syndrome, *COL4A5*, *COL4A4*, *COL4A3*, kidney disease, glomerular basement membrane, hematuria, albuminuria, proteinuria, renal failure, sensorineural deafness, lenticonus, fleck retinopathy, corneal dystrophy, angiotensin-converting enzyme inhibitors

1. Introduction

Alport syndrome is the most frequent hereditary glomerulopathy affecting approximately 1 in 5000–53,000 people. The disease caused by mutations in the *COL4A3*, *COL4A4*, and *COL4A5* genes, which encode the $\alpha3$, $\alpha4$, and $\alpha5$ chains of collagen type IV, a component of the basement membrane of the kidney, the eye, and the inner ear. The syndrome includes progressive nephropathy, ocular abnormalities, and high-tone sensorineural deafness. Clinical features and the prognosis of patients with Alport syndrome are known to depend on mutation type. The most frequent X-linked form of Alport syndrome is caused by *COL4A5* gene defects and detected in 85% of patients. Autosomal recessive inheritance is found in about 15% of patients; it can be caused either by homozygous or compound heterozygous mutations in *COL4A3* or *COL4A4*. Patients who harbor only one pathogenic variant either in *COL4A3* or *COL4A4* gene are usually diagnosed with thin basement membrane nephropathy or autosomal dominant Alport syndrome. Digenic inheritance pattern of Alport syndrome has also been described. Current knowledge and future directions on Alport syndrome will be explored in this review.

2. Alport syndrome: genetic, pathogenesis, clinical presentation, prognosis, and treatment

2.1. Genetic and genotype-phenotype correlations in Alport syndrome

Several clinical cases of patients with hereditary familial congenital hemorrhagic nephritis were published by Arthur C. Alport in 1927. He was the first to recognize the link between nephritis and deafness, and he also noted ocular changes in one of these patients [1].

Alport syndrome (AS) is a multisystem disorder including progressive renal disease, sensori-neural deafness, and eye abnormalities.

Alport syndrome is caused by mutations in the *COL4A3*, *COL4A4*, and *COL4A5* genes, which encode the $\alpha3$, $\alpha4$, and $\alpha5$ chains of collagen type IV, a component of the glomerular basement membrane (GBM) in the kidney.

COL4A5 gene is located on chromosome X. More than 2300 *COL4A5* variants have been described to date [2]. Among the pathogenic variants, about 41% are missense mutations (with overwhelming majority of them being substitutions of glycine in the Gly-Xaa-Yaa triplet of the collagenous domain) which are the most frequent, followed by frameshift, splice site mutations, larger copy number variations, and nonsense mutations [3].

The *COL4A3* and *COL4A4* genes are located on chromosome 2 and share the same promoter (they are transcribed in opposite directions). Among *COL4A3* and *COL4A4* mutations, the distribution of mutation types is similar, in particular, glycine substitutions and missense mutations of other types still dominate. Incidence of pathogenic variants in the two genes is similar [4].

The abovementioned genes are known to have no mutation hotspots; however, some popula-tion-specific founder mutations have been described, e.g., *COL4A5* p.Leu649Arg mutation in the US [5], COL4A5 p.Gly624Asp mutation in the Slovenia, Hungary, and Greece [6–8], and deletion of exons 2–36 of COL4A5 in French Polynesia [9].

The most frequent X-linked form of AS is caused by *COL4A5* gene defects and detected in 85% of patients [10] (80% according to Kashtan [11]). It is dominant and more severe in males, whereas in females, penetrance depends on X chromosome inactivation pattern [12]. Patients demonstrate end-stage renal disease (ESRD) at the age of 8–60 years and usually have microhematuria with macrohematuria episodes from childhood [13]. About 80% of affected families demonstrate sensorineural hearing loss (at least in some patients) and about 50% are characterized by ocular abnormalities [13].

Autosomal recessive inheritance is found in about 15% of patients with their clinical course and ultrastructural changes being similar to those in X-linked form [14]. It can be caused either by homozygous or compound heterozygous mutations in COL4A3 or COL4A4 [15, 16].

Patients who harbor only one pathogenic variant either in COL4A3 or COL4A4 gene are usually diagnosed with thin basement membrane nephropathy (TBMN): benign familial hematuria not progressing to ESRD. It is still disputable if patients bearing only one pathogenic variant in either COL4A3 or COL4A4 gene who suffer from hematuria, lack hearing or ocular abnormalities, and potentially can develop ESRD in late age should be categorized to autosomal dominant AS or TBMN [17].

Digenic inheritance pattern of AS has also been described, which can be caused by two mutations in COL4A3 and COL4A4 genes each (either on the same chromosome or on homologous chromosomes) as well as by a combination of two mutations in COL4A5 and COL4A3 or COL4A4 gene [18].

AS prognosis is known to depend on the mutation type. Associations have been shown both in males with X-linked inheritance and in autosomal recessive form (both sexes). Associations of genotype and phenotype have been extensively studied for the following conditions: age at onset of ESRD, hearing loss, and ocular abnormalities.

The expected ESRD age is similar for the two types of AS and comprises 23–25 years, excluding females with X-linked AS [4]. The risk of ESRD development in patients with X-linked AS by the age of 30 years is 70% in males, whereas only 5% in females; by the age of 40 years: 90 and 10%, respectively [19].

Phenotypic and clinical features in AS are known to depend on mutation type. Among patients with COL4A5 variants, in males, the risk of development of ESRD by 30 years of age is the highest for subjects bearing "severe" mutations (nonsense, frameshift mutations, and multiexon deletions): 90%; lower for subjects bearing splice site variants: 70%; the lowest for patients bearing missense variants: 50% [19]. In females, there is no statistically significant difference neither for age at onset of ESRD nor for presence of hearing or ocular abnormalities [19].

Hearing and ocular abnormalities are also more prevalent in men than in women among X-linked AS subjects [20, 21]. Sensorineural hearing loss by the age of 30 is found in 60% of male patients with missense mutations compared to 90% of patients with mutations of other more severe types (including splice site mutations) [19]. Ocular abnormalities were shown to be 2–4 times less prevalent in males harboring pathogenic missense variants [20, 22, 23].

In patients with autosomal recessive AS, mutation type has similar effect on the clinical prognosis [4], which is significant both for women (unlike for X-linked type) and men.

2.2. Pathogenesis of Alport syndrome

Collagen type IV is composed of six different α chains, which assemble into three different protomers ($\alpha 1\alpha 1\alpha 2$, $\alpha 3\alpha 4\alpha 5$, and $\alpha 5\alpha 5\alpha 6$) with a tissue-specific distribution [24, 25]. The absence of any one of these type IV collagen chains can result in the absence of the whole protomer in the GBM, presumably due to an obligatory association of the three chains in forming the type IV collagen superstructure [26].

The heterotrimers are essential for basement membrane structure and function [26]. The $\alpha3\alpha4\alpha5$ protomer in the GBM is only produced by podocytes [27], that is why podocytes are a key cell type affected by Alport syndrome pathology. The $\alpha1\alpha1\alpha2$ heterotrimer is produced by three cell types in the glomerulus: podocytes, endothelial cells, and mesangial cells [27]. The $\alpha1\alpha1\alpha2$ heterotrimer is ubiquitously distributed in all basement membranes during embryogenesis, and then in the process of development, there is a partial replacement of $\alpha1\alpha1\alpha2$ protomer by $\alpha3\alpha4\alpha5$ heterotrimer in the GBM, lungs, eyes, cochlea, and testes, and by the $\alpha5\alpha5\alpha6$ heterotrimer in skin, smooth muscle cells, kidney's Bowman capsules, and esophagus [28]. This substitution of collagen type IV heterotrimers leads to mechanical stability of basement membrane, as the $\alpha1\alpha1\alpha2$ chains are highly susceptible to endoproteolysis. In AS, assembly of the $\alpha3\alpha4\alpha5$ heterotrimer does not occur, resulting in decreased mechanical stability and splitting of the GBM, as well as other tissue-specific pathological changes.

The detailed pathogenetic mechanisms leading to progression of AS are not clear. As the GBM is a key component of the filtration barrier, patients with AS develop proteinuria [29] as a result of altered podocyte orientation, podocyte effacement, and disruption of slit diaphragms. However, interactions between integrins and the laminin $\alpha5\beta2\gamma1$ heterotrimer could disrupt the actin cytoskeleton and activate signaling mechanisms that result in an increase in matrix metalloproteinase expression and massive accumulation of extracellular matrix [25] as well as kidney fibrosis due to fibroblast formation by epithelial-mesenchymal transition, initiated as a physiological repair of injury response [30]. Invasion of mesangial filopodia may be responsible for deposition of the extracellular molecules in Alport GBM [31–33]. These changes could lead to progression of glomerulosclerosis, nephron loss, and hypertension. Increasing deposition of extracellular matrix and laminin $\alpha5$, upregulation of matrix metalloproteinase has been shown in the stria vascularis of ear in vivo.

Ultrastructural studies have demonstrated that the fundamental lesion of AS involves the GBM [29, 34]. The typical changes of GBM in AS are its thickening, splitting, and fragmentation of the lamina densa with formation of a characteristic "basket weave" pattern. The lesions may be focal (in the early stages of the disease) or widespread (in the late stages). The thinning or irregular appearance of the GBM (an alternation of thickening and thinning) is the prevalent changes in children with AS. Diffuse thinning of the GBM as the only morphological changes may be observed in 10–20% of patients with Alport syndrome, explaining why patients with thin basal membranes may have an unfavorable prognosis. Sometimes, it is possible to see the focal ruptures of the GBM and its reparation due to the synthesis of the new material of the glomerular basement membrane [35]. The light microscopy changes are not specific and vary from the normal renal tissue appearance or minimal glomerular changes in the early stages of the disease to focal mesangial proliferation, focal and segmental thickening of the capillary walls, and focal/global glomerulosclerosis in the late stages of the AS. These changes are associated with nonspecific tubulointerstitial lesions including foci of lipid-laden foam cells. Conventional immunofluorescence detects nothing or only faint or focal deposits of IgG, IgM, or complement C3.

The distribution of the different chains of collagen type IV in the basement membranes is very important for diagnosis of AS and especially for X-linked transmission's recognition.

Normally, *COL4A5* is expressed in the glomerular basement membranes, and the α5(IV) chain defect due to *COL4A5* mutation (absence or abnormal structure of α5(IV)) impairs protomer assembly and the normal collagen IV network formation. Immunohistological analysis reveals abnormal distribution of the α5(IV) chain in about two-thirds of patients with X-linked AS: in male patients, the α5(IV) antigen is not detected in the glomerular, capsular, and distal tubular basement membranes, while in female patients, the α5(IV) antigen has a discontinuous distribution. In addition, there is a lack of the α3(IV) and α4(IV) chains which participate in the α3α4α5(IV)-α3α4α5(IV) network formation. At the same time, the α1(IV) and α2(IV) chains normally confining to the mesangium and the subendothelial aspect of the GBM are widely expressed throughout the glomerular basement membrane in these patients. This immunohistological picture is typical for the fetal kidneys. But approximately, one-third of patients with AS do not have marked changes in the renal expression of α(IV) chains. The immunohistochemical picture is usually consistent within the family and correlates with the severity of the clinicopathological features of the disease [25, 36].

The distribution of α(IV) chains is also abnormal in skin basement membrane: the absence of the α5(IV) and the associated α6(IV) chains from the epidermal basement membrane is typical for male patients with X-linked AS and can be detected in about two-thirds of male patients. Observation of normal patterns of α5(IV) and α6(IV) localization does not facilitate definitive diagnosis in females because of the segmental distribution of the chains.

The peculiar immunohistochemical distribution pattern of α3(IV) to α6(IV) chains is observed in the skin and kidneys of most patients with autosomal recessive AS [31, 32, 35] and is characterized by the absence of α3, α4, and α5(IV) chains from the GBM contrasting with the persistence of α5(IV) chains in Bowman's capsules, collecting ducts, and epidermal basement membranes. These findings show that in autosomal recessive Alport patients, the expression of α5(IV) chains is defective only in those basement membranes in which the three chains are associated within the α3α4α5(IV)-α3α4α5(IV) network.

Expression of mutant collagen type IV results in splitting of the GBM, podocyte effacement, glomerulosclerosis, kidney fibrosis, and ESRD progression.

Men who are hemizygous for mutations in *COL4A5* causing X-linked AS have similar clinical presentation and prognosis to individuals homozygous for *COL4A3* and *COL4A4* mutations causing autosomal recessive AS. The median age of ESRD onset in untreated male patients with X-linked AS has been reported to be 22 years (range 7–39 years) [37, 38]. But, owing to imprinting (random inactivation on the two X chromosomes in female individuals) [39], female carriers of *COL4A5* mutations causing X-linked AS may have a higher risk of ESRD than do individuals who are heterozygous for autosomal recessive mutations in *COL4A3* and *COL4A4*.

2.3. Clinical presentation of Alport syndrome

The diagnosis of AS should be suspected in patients with family glomerular hematuria and with family history of renal failure. Children with AS syndrome can usually be diagnosed with mild hematuria with or no episodic macrohematuria and low-grade proteinuria. As the disease progresses, patients gradually develop severe proteinuria and progressive renal failure. Irrespective of the mode of inheritance of the disorder, proteinuria indicates an increased risk of progressive renal disease, even in heterozygous carriers. Changes in the GBM that are pathognomonic for AS include splitting and enlargement of the GBM and podocyte effacement.

There are several clinical stages in the development of glomerulopathy in AS:

Stage 0: microscopic hematuria (albumin/creatinine rate <30 mg/g/day).

Stage 1: microalbuminuria (albumin/creatinine rate = 30–300 mg/g/day).

Stage 2: gross proteinuria (albumin/creatinine rate >300 mg/g/day).

Stage 3: impaired renal function (glomerular filtration rate <60 ml/min/1.73 m^2).

Stage 4: end-stage renal disease.

Diagnosis of AS can be made in most patients after a clinical examination on the basis of the typical symptoms including kidney, ear, and eye.

The sensorineural hearing loss in AS, which primarily affects high tones, occurs in 30–50% of relatives with renal disease. The severity of auditory and renal features does not correlate. The molecular defects that underlie the otopathology in this disease remain poorly understood. An animal model of X-linked AS showed complete absence of the α3α4α5 network in the inner ear, suggesting that collagen type IV is vital to cochlear function as well as renal function. The generation of radial tension of the spiral ligament on the basilar membrane via the extracellular matrix is necessary for reception of high-frequency sound. The lateral aspect of the spiral ligament is populated by tension fibroblasts expressing nonmuscle myosin and α-smooth muscle actin [40]. On the basis of the foregoing, it was assumed that in AS, the loss of the α3α4α5 network eventually weakens the interaction of fibroblasts with their extracellular matrix, resulting in reduced tension on the basilar membrane and the inability to respond to high-frequency sounds [40]. Findings in Alport mice suggest that the hearing loss may arise from dysfunction of the stria vascularis mediated through endothelin-1 [40, 41].

The ocular manifestations in Alport syndrome patients are caused by loss of the collagen IV α3α4α5 network in basement membranes of the eyes due to mutations which lead to basement membrane thinning, lamellation, and a decrease in its mechanical stability. Most of the ocular features in AS do not lead to a visual impairment, but they have diagnostic and prognostic value: in some cases, the ocular symptoms suggest the mode of inheritance and the likelihood of early-onset renal failure. Such ocular features as central and peripheral retinopathy and lenticonus are typical for AS, and their presence confirms the diagnosis.

Anterior lenticonus can be detected in half of men (not women) with X-linked Alport syndrome. And its presence is associated with early-onset renal failure. The symptom is often found in autosomal recessive AS regardless of the patient's sex, and therefore, the presence of lenticonus in women with AS most likely indicates an autosomal recessive mode of disease inheritance [41, 42]. Lenticonus is the consequence of the conical protrusion of the lens anteriorly through the thinnest part of the capsule [43]; sometimes, the mechanical weakness of the capsule due to the absence of the $\alpha3\alpha4\alpha5$ network can lead to its spontaneous ruptures and secondary cataract developments [44, 45]. After cataract formation, lenticonus ceases to progress [46]. Posterior lenticonus is less common in patients with AS. Lenticonus is usually found in early middle-age patients with renal failure. The patients complain a progressive difficulty in focusing due to of their abnormal lens shape. The presence of an oil droplet sign on direct ophthalmoscopy or slit-lamp examination confirms the diagnosis. Visual symptoms progress with a time, and most patients eventually require surgery. The treatment for both symptomatic lenticonus and cataract includes the lens removal and intraocular lens implantation.

The central or perimacular fleck retinopathy and peripheral coalescing fleck retinopathy are common retinal abnormalities in patients with AS. The other retinal changes include manifestations of temporal thinning [47, 48]: lamellar and giant macular hole, a lozenge, loss of the foveal reflex, disturbances of foveal pigmentation, including a bull's eye or vitelliform maculopathy [48, 49]. Central fleck retinopathy is present in 60% of men and at least 15% of women with X-linked AS and 50% of individuals with recessive disease [50]. It is more common with early-onset renal failure and lenticonus [47]. The central retinopathy varies from scattered whitish-yellow dots and flecks to a dense, almost confluent annulus around the region of temporal retinal thinning. The fleck retinopathy is associated with an abnormal inner limiting membrane. Thinning of the inner limiting membrane/nerve fiber layer may interfere with the nutrition of the overlying cells, removal of debris, and maintenance of the watertight barrier. The central retinopathy is best seen with color photographs and red-free images centered on the macula. Specialized tests of retinal function, such as electroretinogram and electrooculogram, are normal or nearly normal. The peripheral fleck retinopathy is the most common retinal abnormality, occurring in most men and 25% of women with X-linked AS and most individuals with recessive disease [47, 48]. The asymmetric patches of confluent flecks are characteristic signs of peripheral retinopathy [50]. The appearance on optical coherence tomography (OCT) and fleck location in relation to the blood vessels suggests that their formation is related to pathological changes of the retinal pigment epithelium/Bruch's membrane. The peripheral retinopathy is a very important diagnostic and prognostic symptom of AS associated with early-onset renal failure, central retinopathy, and lenticonus. But the peripheral retinopathy can also be present in women with X-linked AS who have normal renal function [47]. The peripheral retinopathy is best seen on ophthalmic examination or with retinal photographs that extend beyond the standard views into the periphery and with red-free retinal images. Temporal retinal thinning is very common in men and women with X-linked AS, and in patients with recessive disease [41, 42, 47, 48]. The lozenge, dull macular reflex, foveopathy, and lamellar and macular holes all affect the temporal retina and reflect retinal thinning of both the inner limiting membrane and Bruch's membrane. Thinning is confirmed with retinal thickness measurements on OCT. However, thinning is common in all forms of Alport syndrome and less sensitive diagnostically than a peripheral retinopathy. Hypopigmentation occurred in Alport syndrome is often not diagnosed. It is usually present along with perimacular flecks or other ocular features and does not lead to the visual impairment. Severe forms, such as a bull's eye or vitelliform retinopathy, may be occasionally found. Lamellar, partial-thickness macular holes, and giant macular holes lamellar are uncommon in patients with X-linked and autosomal recessive AS. This sign is unspecific for

AS. But in AS, the macular holes are larger (giant holes) and occur at a younger age than the spontaneous holes in patients who do not have AS. Holes may be asymmetric, unilateral, or bilateral. Beginning with multiple small defects, they hollow out from the surface of the inner limiting membrane in the consequence of accelerated passage of fluid through the defective Bruch's membrane, and followed by microcysts formation due to membrane breaking [50]. Patients with macular holes suffer from metamorphopsia (where straight lines are distorted) and impairment of central vision. In some patients, holes only become evident when there is no improvement in vision after surgery for lenticonus. Lamellar holes might be overlooked by retinal photographs; the OCT is required for their demonstration. Holes in AS do not respond well to surgical closure and often lead to a permanent loss of vision.

Posterior polymorphous corneal dystrophy and macular hole are rare but also suggest the Alport syndrome. Corneal disease is recognized infrequently in Alport syndrome. Erosions result from an abnormal Bowman's membrane in the corneal subepithelium and posterior polymorphous corneal dystrophy from an abnormal Descemet's membrane in the subendothelium [41]. The affected membranes lack the collagen IV $\alpha3\alpha4\alpha5$ network, are weak, and adhere poorly to the epithelium, endothelium, and underlying stroma. Superficial corneal erosions occur in 10% of patients, but they are intermittent and hence. Their onset may precede the diagnosis of AS and is often in the late teenage years. They typically occur in individuals with early-onset renal failure and other extrarenal features. Posterior polymorphous corneal dystrophy is rare and more serious than the corneal erosions. Patients may be asymptomatic or have photophobia, watering, and grittiness. The diagnosis is based on high-resolution anterior segment OCT, slit-lamp biomicroscopy, specular microscopy, or in vivo confocal microscopy: there are multiple clusters of vesicles ("doughnuts") or bands ("snail tracks") at the posterior corneal surface. The vesicles result from vacuolar degeneration of dying cells or multilayered epithelial cell protuberances from Descemet's membrane. Treatment is usually symptomatic; sometimes, the dystrophy progresses, and corneal transplantation is required.

Ocular features are less sensitive but more specific than hearing loss in diagnostic of AS, because hearing loss occurs also in other inherited renal diseases and in dialysis patients. In addition, ocular symptoms may help distinguish between X-linked and autosomal recessive inheritance. Central retinopathy, lenticonus, and macular hole are rare in women with X-linked AS. The presence of any of these futures in a woman with hematuria leads to suspected autosomal recessive AS. Furthermore, revealed peripheral retinopathy in the mother of a boy with hematuria indicates the diagnosis of AS and also X-linked inheritance of the disease. Some ocular features have a prognostic value because they are associated with early-onset renal failure. Thus, central retinopathy and lenticonus usually indicate the onset of renal failure before the age of 30 years. Therefore, it is important to conduct a thorough ophthalmologic examination (slit-lamp examination, retinal photography, and OCT) in assessing patients with suspected AS. These tests are acceptable to patients, noninvasive, inexpensive, and widely available.

Other features of Alport syndrome include gastroesophageal leiomyomatosis and vascular abnormalities. Gastroesophageal leiomyomatosis is a very rare pathology characterized by benign nodular tumors with smooth muscle cells origin. The condition clinically presents by dysphagia. Leiomyomatosis can also affect the tracheobronchial tree and the genital tract. Leiomyomatosis in AS is a consequence of a large deletion in the *COL4A5* and *COL4A6* genes, which encode collagen α5 (IV) or α5α6 (IV) chains in smooth muscle cells of the gastroesophageal tract [51, 52]. The α5 and α6 chains of type IV collagen are also found in the basement membranes surrounding vascular smooth muscle cells in the intima and media of aorta and other arteries in mice model [53]. Seki et al. [53] believed that α5 and α6 chains of type IV collagen in the basement membranes may have particular function in the arteries which are required to tolerate strong pulse and blood pressure such as the aorta. AS is associated with aortic abnormalities including aortic dilatation, ruptured ascending aortic aneurysm, aortic dissection, aortic insufficiency, and bicuspid aortic valve and coronary artery pathology including spontaneous coronary artery dissection in male patients [54–56].

Furthermore, patients with AS and mitral valve prolapse or ventricular septal defects and ruptured intracranial and coronary artery aneurysms have also been described [54, 57]. Therefore, the vascular imaging techniques could be included in the examination of patients with AS, especially in cases of family history of vascular abnormalities.

2.4. Differential diagnosis of Alport syndrome

In cases where the diagnosis of AS was not confirmed by clinical workup, morphology, or genetic test, other diseases with similar symptoms should be considered. A combination of kidney pathology and hearing loss can be associated with mutations of gene encoding mitochondrial and cytoskeletal proteins, ion channels, and receptors.

Patients with mitochondriopathy associated with mutations in the *COQ6* gene develop early-onset steroid-resistant nephrotic syndrome and sensorineural deafness [58]. The mutation leads to deficiency of ubiquinone biosynthesis monooxygenase COQ6 protein, localized in the Golgi apparatus of the stria vascularis and glomerular podocytes, and to upregulation of proapoptotic factors [58].

Alström syndrome is characterized by a defect of the primary cilium that is caused by mutations in *ALMS1* and leads to renal failure, sensorineural deafness in young adulthood, and vision loss in adulthood [59].

MYH-9-related disease should be considered in patients presenting with proteinuria and thrombocytopenia [60]. *MYH-9*-related disease (the gene for the heavy chain of nonmuscle myosin IIA) is a rare inherited autosomal dominant condition characterized by progressive nephritis (39%), macrothrombocytopenia (100%), Dohle-like leukocyte inclusions (100%), high-tone sensorineural deafness (49%), and cataract (54%) [60, 61]. Renal disease ranged from microscopic hematuria to end-stage renal failure necessitating dialysis and kidney transplantation. The most striking difference between hearing loss in *MYH-9*-related disease (or Fechtner syndrome) and that in AS was that the vast majority of hearing disorders in the latter occur in male patients. Hearing loss in *MYH-9*-related disease develops from the second decade of life and progresses slowly with several episodes of sudden deafness [60]. Renal biopsy findings are consistent with those of AS. Chronic renal failure can occur at a young age in patients with *MYH-9*-related disease.

A recent report described a *COL4A1* frameshift mutation in a family with autosomal dominant hematuria, GBM thinning, kidney cysts, and progressive kidney disease [62, 63]. The syndrome is characterized by hereditary angiopathy with retinal tortuosities, aneurysms, muscular cramps, and nephropathy manifesting as hematuria or cysts (HANAC). As such, investigation of patients with unexplained hematuria should include a search for extrarenal symptoms of HANAC, especially retinal abnormalities.

2.5. Renal prognosis

The expected ESRD age is similar for the males with X-linked and patients with autosomal recessive AS and comprises 23–25 years [4]. The risk of ESRD development in patients with X-linked AS by the age of 20 years is 70% in males, whereas only 5% in females; by the age of 40 years: 90 and 10%, respectively [19]. For many years, female members of Alport families who had hematuria were considered to be carriers who were not at risk for ESRD, despite reports of ESRD in female Alport patients. But review of clinical outcomes of nearly 300 girls and women with confirmed heterozygous *COL4A5* mutations showed that 12 and 30% of female have the probability of developing ESRD before the age of 40 and 60 years, respectively [19]. The 95% of heterozygous females had hematuria, the 75%—proteinuria; in addition, it was found that the proteinuria increased the risk of ESRD.

Patients with heterozygous mutations compared to patients with mutations in both alleles of *COL4A3* or *COL4A4* (autosomal recessive Alport syndrome) or hemizygous mutations in *COL4A5* (males with X-linked Alport syndrome) usually have milder renal involvement with late ESRD development and do not have extrarenal manifestations (ocular changes and hearing loss). But, lifetime risk of ESRD in heterozygous patients is higher than in the general population [64].

AS accounted for 0.5% of all cases of ESRD and was found to be associated with superior dialysis patient survival, superior posttransplant patient survival, and potentially superior renal allograft survival to matched controls with other causes of ESRD [65–67]. An incidence rate of anti-GBM antibody disease after kidney transplantation comprises 1–5% [65–67].

2.6. Treatment of Alport syndrome

Early diagnosis of AS is important, since therapeutic blockade of the renin-angiotensin-aldosterone system can slow the progression to ESRD depending on the stage of the disease when therapy is initiated. Angiotensin-converting enzyme (ACE) inhibitors are not a specific therapy for AS. The antihypertensive and antiproteinuric properties of ACE inhibitors lead to their nephroprotective effect. The animal models of AS have shown a major role of altered composition of the GBM and of podocytes (their cytoskeleton and their collagen receptors) with activation of profibrotic factors in disease progression [32, 33]. ACE inhibitors seem to be able to downregulate profibrotic factors independently from blood pressure and the amount of proteinuria in the Alport animal model [68].

The Alport Syndrome Research Collaborative recommends use of ACE inhibitors in all affected individuals with microalbuminuria or proteinuria, and underlines the importance of using standardized dosing regimens and monitoring microalbuminuria during the treatment [69]. The ACE inhibitor ramipril is recommended as the first-line therapy; in cases of adverse effects associated with use of ramipril, the treatment with angiotensin-1-receptor antagonists will be recommended [69, 70]. The Alport Syndrome Research Collaborative guidelines suggest, therefore, that therapy with ACE inhibitors can be considered as early as stages 0 and 1 of the disease [69].

The age at progression from microalbuminuria to proteinuria in children with Alport syndrome is an important prognostic marker—the earlier this transition occurs, the worse the prognosis [71].

Currently, the only recruiting trial is the prospective, randomized placebo-controlled EARLY PRO-TECT Alport trial, enrolling pediatric patients with stages 0 and 1 Alport syndrome [72]. The goal of this trial is to clarify whether an early start of therapy delays renal failure more effectively than later onset of therapy and, above all, whether therapy in the early stages of Alport syndrome is safe. The trial will also investigate a potential protective effect of ramipril against the hearing loss as a secondary end point [72]. It seems to be very important because currently there are no therapies that can prevent the ocular changes or hearing loss development and progression in patients with AS.

Studies in animal models have revealed many potential new therapies for use in Alport syndrome: inhibitors of proinflammatory factors (for example, TGF-β1 and MMPs) [73, 74]; statins [75]; BX471 (a chemokine receptor-1 blocker) [76]; and upregulation of the expression of bone morphogenetic protein 7 [77]. A phase II study of antimicroRNA-21 treatment of patients with Alport syndrome 18 years of age or older with glomerular filtration rates of 45–90 ml/min/1.73 m^2 will be start; its primary goal will be determining the glomerular filtration rate decline during therapy [78]. In transgenic Alport mice, antimicroRNA-21 treatment reduced glomerular inflammation and impaired renal fibrotic pathways. A phase II/III study of the efficacy and safety of bardoxolone methyl for Alport syndrome patients with chronic kidney disease (CARDINAL) has been started [79].

3. Conclusion

Alport syndrome is a multisystem hereditary disorder characterized by progressive renal disease, sensorineural deafness, and eye abnormalities. Diagnosis of AS can be made on the basis of the typical symptoms, renal morphology, and/or genetic tests. Early diagnosis of Alport syndrome is very important, since therapeutic blockade of the renin-angiotensin-aldosterone system can slow the progression to ESRD.

Conflict of interest

The authors declare no conflict of interest.

Appendices and Nomenclature

AS   Alport syndrome

ACE   angiotensin-converting enzyme

GBM   glomerular basement membrane

ESRD   end-stage renal disease

OCT   optical coherence tomography

TBMN   thin basement membrane nephropathy

Author details

Marina Aksenova* and Lev Shagam

*Address all correspondence to: maksyonova@pedklin.ru

Y.Veltischev Research and Clinical Institute for Pediatrics at the Pirogov Russian National Research Medical University, Moscow, Russia

References

[1] Alport AC. Hereditary familial congenital haemorrhagic nephritis. British Medical Journal. 1927;**1**:504-506. PMID: 20773074

[2] Leiden Open Variation database, gene COL4A5. [Internet]. Available from: https://databases.lovd.nl/shared/transcripts/COL4A5 [Accessed: 2018.04.28]

[3] Hertz J, Thomassen M, Storey H, Flinter F. Clinical utility gene card for: Alport syndrome. EJHG. 2012;**6**:20. DOI: 10.1038/ejhg.2011.237

[4] Savige J, Storey H, Il Cheong H, Gyung Kang H, et al. X-linked and autosomal recessive Alport syndrome: Pathogenic variant features and further genotype-phenotype correlations. PLoS One. 2016;**11**(9):e0161802. DOI: 10.1371/journal.pone.0161802

[5] Barker D, Pruchno C, Jiang X, Atkin C, Stone E, et al. A mutation causing Alport syndrome with tardive hearing loss is common in the western United States. American Journal of Human Genetics. 1996;**6**(58):1157-1165. PMID: 8651292

[6] Demosthenous P, Voskarides K, Stylianou K, Hadjigavriel M, Arsali M, et al. X-linked Alport syndrome in Hellenic families: Phenotypic heterogeneity and mutations near interruptions of the collagen domain in COL4A5. Clinical Genetics. 2012;**3**(81):240-248. DOI: 10.1111/j.1399-0004.2011.01647

[7] Kovács G, Kalmár T, Endreffy E, Ondrik Z, Iványi B, et al. Efficient targeted next generation sequencing-based workflow for differential diagnosis of Alport-related disorders. PLoS One. 2016;3(11):e0149241. DOI: 10.1371/journal.pone.0149241

[8] Slajpah M, Gorinsek B, Berginc G, Vizjak A, Ferluga D, et al. Sixteen novel mutations identified in COL4A3, COL4A4, and COL4A5 genes in Slovenian families with Alport syndrome and benign familial hematuria. Kidney International. 2007;12(71):1287-1295. DOI: 10.1038/sj.ki.5002221

[9] Arrondel C, Deschênes G, Le Meur Y, Viau A, Cordonnier C, et al. A large tandem duplication within the COL4A5 gene is responsible for the high prevalence of Alport syndrome in French Polynesia. Kidney International. 2004;6(65):2030-2040. DOI: 10.1111/j.1523-1755.2004.00622.x

[10] Martin P, Heiskari N, Zhou J, Leinonen A, Tumelius T, et al. High mutation detection rate in the COL4A5 collagen gene in suspected Alport syndrome using PCR and direct DNA sequencing. JASN. 1998;12(9):2291-2301. PMID:9848783

[11] Kashtan C. Alport syndrome: Facts and opinions. F1000Research. 2017;6:50. DOI: 10.12688/f1000research.9636.1

[12] Rheault M. Women and Alport syndrome. Pediatric Nephrology. 2012;1(27):41-46. DOI: 10.1007/s00467-011-1836-7

[13] Pierides A, Voskarides V, Kkolou M, Hadjigavriel M, Deltas C. X-linked, COL4A5 hypomorphic Alport mutations such as G624D and P628L may only exhibit thin basement membrane nephropathy with microhematuria and late onset kidney failure. Hippokratia. 2013;3(17):207-213. PMC3872455

[14] Haas M. Alport syndrome and thin glomerular basement membrane nephropathy: A practical approach to diagnosis. Archives of Pathology & Laboratory Medicine. 2009;2(133):224-232. DOI: 10.1043/1543-2165(2006)130[699:TGBMNI]2.0.CO;2

[15] Lemmink H, Hughes A, Hill C, Smeets H, Doherty C, et al. Mutations in the type IV collagen alpha 3 (COL4A3) gene in autosomal recessive Alport syndrome. Human Molecular Genetics. 1994;8(3):1269-1273. PMID:7987301

[16] Mochizuki T, Lemmink H, Mariyama M, Antignac C, Gubler M, et al. Identification of mutations in the alpha 3(IV) and alpha 4(IV) collagen genes in autosomal recessive Alport syndrome. Nature Genetics. 1994;1(8):77-81. DOI: 10.1038/ng0994-77

[17] Miner J, Baigent C, Flinter F, Gross O, Judge P, et al. The 2014 international workshop on Alport syndrome. Kidney International. 2014;4(86):679-684. DOI: 10.1038/ki.2014.229

[18] Mencarelli M, Heidet L, Storey H, van Geel M, Knebelmann B, et al. Evidence of digenic inheritance in Alport syndrome. Journal of Medical Genetics. 2015;3(52):163-174. DOI: 10.1136/jmedgenet-2014-102822

[19] Jais J, Knebelmann B, Giatras J, De Marchi M, Rizzoni G, et al. X-linked Alport syndrome: Natural history and genotype-phenotype correlations in girls and women belonging to

195 families: A "European Community Alport syndrome concerted action" study. JASN. 2003;**10**(14):2603-2610. DOI: 10.1097/01.ASN.0000090034.71205.74

[20] Tan R, Colville D, Wang Y, Rigby L, Savige J. Alport retinopathy results from "severe" COL4A5 mutations and predicts early renal failure. CJASN. 2010;**1**(5):34-38. DOI: 10. 2215/CJN.01030209

[21] Nabais Sá M, Sampaio S, Oliveira A, Alves S, Moura C, et al. Collagen type IV-related nephropathies in Portugal: Pathogenic COL4A5 mutations and clinical characterization of 22 families. Clinical Genetics. 2015;**5**(88):462-467. DOI: 10.1111/cge.12522

[22] Bekheirnia M, Reed B, Gregory M, McFann K, Shamshirsaz A, et al. Genotype-phenotype correlation in X-linked Alport syndrome. JASN. 2010;**5**(21):876-883. DOI: 10.1681/ASN. 2009070784

[23] Gross O, Netzer K, Lambrecht R, Seibold S, Weber M. Meta-analysis of genotype-phenotype correlation in X-linked Alport syndrome: Impact on clinical counseling. Nephrology, Dialysis, Transplantation. 2002;**7**(17):1218-1227. PMID: 12105244

[24] Khoshnoodi J, Pedchenko V, Hudson B. Mammalian collagen IV. Microscopy Research and Technique. 2008;**71**:357-370. DOI: 10.3109/03008207.2013.867337

[25] Hudson B. The molecular basis of Goodpasture and Alport syndromes: Beacons for the discovery of the collagen IV family. JASN. 2004;**15**:2514-2527. DOI: 10.1097/01.ASN. 0000141462.00630.76

[26] Poschl E, Schlötzer-Schrehardt U, Brachvogel B, Saito K, Ninomiya Y, et al. Collagen IV is essential for basement membrane stability but dispensable for initiation of its assembly during early development. Development. 2004;**131**:1619-1628. DOI: 10.1242/dev.01037

[27] Abrahamson D, Hudson B, Stroganova L, Borza D, John P. Cellular origins of type IV collagen networks in developing glomeruli. JASN. 2009;**20**:1471-1479. DOI: 10.1681/ ASN.2008101086

[28] Ninomiya Y, Kagawa M, Iyama K, Naito I, Kishiro Y, et al. Differential expression of two basement membrane collagen genes, COL4A6 and COL4A5, demonstrated by immuno-fluorescence staining using peptide-specific monoclonal antibodies. The Journal of Cell Biology. 1995;**130**:1219-1229. PMC2120565

[29] Hamano Y, Grunkemeyer J, Sudhakar A, Zeisberg M, Cosgrove D, et al. Determinants of vascular permeability in the kidney glomerulus. The Journal of Biological Chemistry. 2010;**277**:31154-31162. DOI: 10.1074/jbc.M204806200

[30] Zeisberg M, Neilson E. Mechanisms of tubulointerstitial fibrosis. JASN. 2010;**21**:1819-1834. DOI: 10.1681/ASN.2010080793

[31] Van Agtmael T, Bruckner-Tuderman L. Basement membranes and human disease. Cell and Tissue Research. 2010;**339**:167-188. DOI: 10.1007/s00441-009-0866-y

[32] Wiradjaja F, DiTommaso T, Smyth I. Basement membranes in development and disease. Birth Defects Research. Part C, Embryo Today. 2010;**90**:8-31. DOI: 10.1002/bdrc.20172

[33] Kruegel J, Miosge N. Basement membrane components are key players in specialized extracellular matrices. Cellular and Molecular Life Sciences. 2010;67:2879-2895. DOI: 10.1007/s00018-010-0367-x

[34] Miner J. Organogenesis of the kidney glomerulus: Focus on the glomerular basement membrane. Organogenesis. 2011;7:75-82. DOI: 10.4161/org.7.2.15275

[35] Cosgrove D. Glomerular pathology in Alport syndrome: A molecular perspective. Pediatric Nephrology. 2012;27:885-890. DOI: 10.1007/s00467-011-1868-z

[36] Gross O, Beirowski B, Harvey S, McFadden C, Chen D, et al. DDR1-deficient mice show localized subepithelial GBM thickening with focal loss of slit diaphragms and proteinuria. Kidney International. 2004;66:102-111. DOI: 10.1111/j.1523-1755.2004.00712.x

[37] Flinter F, Cameron J, Chantler C, Houston I, Bobrow M. Genetics of classic Alport's syndrome. Lancet. 1988;2:1005-1007. DOI: PMID:2902439

[38] Gross O, Licht C, Anders HJ, Hoppe B, Beck B, et al. Early angiotensin-converting enzyme inhibition in Alport syndrome delays renal failure and improves life expectancy. Kidney International. 2012;81:494-501. DOI: 10.1038/ki.2011.407

[39] Migeon B. X inactivation, female mosaicism, and sex differences in renal diseases. JASN. 2008;19:2052-2059. DOI: 10.1681/ASN.2008020198

[40] Meehan D, Delimont D, Dufek B, Zallocchi M, Phillips G, et al. Endothelin-1 mediated induction of extracellular matrix genes in strial marginal cells underlies strial pathology in Alport mice. Hearing Research. 2016;341:100-108. DOI: 10.1016/j.heares.2016.08.003

[41] Colville D, Savige J. Alport syndrome. A review of the ocular manifestations. Ophthalmic Genetics. 1997;18:161-173. DOI: 10.3109/13816819709041431

[42] Colville D, Savige J, Morfis M, Ellis J, Kerr P, et al. Ocular manifestations of autosomal recessive Alport syndrome. Ophthalmic Genetics. 1997;18:119-128. PMID9361309

[43] Ohkubo S, Takeda H, Higashide T, Ito M, Sakurai M, Shirao Y, et al. Immunohistochemical and molecular genetic evidence for type IV collagen $\alpha 5$ chain abnormality in the anterior lenticonus associated with Alport syndrome. Archives of Ophthalmology. 2003;121: 846-850. DOI: 10.1001/archopht.121.6.846

[44] Citirik M, Batman C, Men G, Tuncel M, Zilelioglu O. Electron microscopic examination of the anterior lens capsule in a case of Alport's syndrome. Clinical & Experimental Optometry. 2007;90:367-370. DOI: 10.1111/j.1444-0938.2007.00134.x

[45] Choi J, Na K, Bae S, Roh G. Anterior lens capsule abnormalities in Alport syndrome. Korean Journal of Ophthalmology. 2005;19:84-89. DOI: 10.3341/kjo.2005.19.1.84

[46] Wilson M, Trivedi R, Biber J, Golub R. Anterior capsule rupture and subsequent cataract formation in Alport syndrome. Journal of AAPOS. 2006;10:182-183. DOI: 10.1016/j.jaapos.2005.09.008

[47] Tan R, Colville D, Wang Y, Rigby L, Savige J. Alport retinopathy results from "severe" COL4A5 mutations and predicts early renal failure. CJASN. 2010;5:34-38. DOI: 10.2215/CJN.01030209

[48] Fawzi A, Lee N, Eliott D, Song J, Stewart J. Retinal findings in patients with Alport syndrome: Expanding the clinical spectrum. The British Journal of Ophthalmology. 2009;**93**:1606-1611. DOI: 10.1136/bjo.2009.158089

[49] Savige J, Liu J, DeBuc D, Handa J, Hageman G, et al. Retinal basement membrane abnormalities and the retinopathy of Alport syndrome. Investigative Ophthalmology & Visual Science. 2010;**51**:1621-1627. DOI: 10.1167/iovs.08-3323

[50] Walia S, Fishman G, Kapur R. Flecked-retina syndromes. Ophthalmic Genetics. 2009; **30**:69-75. DOI: 10.1080/13816810802654516

[51] Zhang X, Zhou J, Reeders S, Tryggvason K. Structure of the human type IV collagen COL4A6 gene, which is mutated in Alport syndrome-associated leiomyomatosis. Genomics. 1996;**33**:473-479. DOI: 10.1006/geno.1996.0222

[52] Miner J. Alport syndrome with diffuse leiomyomatosis. When and when not? The American Journal of Pathology. 1999;**154**:1633-1635. DOI: 10.1016/S0002-9440(10)65417-X

[53] Seki T, Naito I, Oohashi T, Sado Y, Ninomiya Y. Differential expression of type IV collagen isoforms, $\alpha5(IV)$ and $\alpha6(IV)$ chains, in basement membranes surrounding smooth muscle cells. Histochemistry and Cell Biology. 1998;**110**(4):359-366. PMID:9792414

[54] Kashtan C, Segal Y, Flinter F, Makanjuola D, Gan J-S, Watnick T. Aortic abnormalities in males with Alport syndrome. Nephrology, Dialysis, Transplantation. 2010;**25**(11): 3554-3560. DOI: 10.1093/ndt/gfq271

[55] D'ıez-Del Hoyo F, Sanz-Ruiz R, D'ıez-Villanueva P, Núñez-García A, Casado-Plasencia A, et al. A novel cardiovascular presentation of Alport syndrome: Spontaneous coronary artery dissection. International Journal of Cardiology. 2014;**177**(3):e133-e134. DOI: 10.1016/j.ijcard.2014.09.065

[56] Earl T, Khan L, Hagau D, Fernandez A. The spectrum of aortic pathology in Alport syndrome: A case report and review of the literature. American Journal of Kidney Diseases. 2012;**60**(5):821-822. DOI: 10.1053/j.ajkd.2012.06.024

[57] Trąbka-Zawicki A, Zmudka K. Giant aneurysms of coronary arteries accidentally discovered following out of hospital cardiac arrest. Kardiologia Polska. 2013;**71**(8):885. DOI: 10.5603/KP.2013.0212

[58] Heeringa S, Chernin G, Chaki M, Zhou W, Sloan A, et al. COQ6 mutations in human patients produce nephrotic syndrome with sensorineural deafness. The Journal of Clinical Investigation. 2011;**121**:2013-2024. DOI: 10.1172/JCI45693

[59] Girard D, Petrovsky N. Alström syndrome: Insights into the pathogenesis of metabolic disorders. Nature Reviews. Endocrinology. 2011;**7**:77-88. DOI: 10.1038/nrendo.2010.210

[60] Ishida M, Mori Y, Ota N, Inaba T, Kunishima S. Association of a novel in-frame deletion mutation of the MYH9 gene with end-stage renal failure: Case report and review of the literature. Clinical Nephrology. 2013;**80**(3):218-222. DOI: 10.5414/CN107237

[61] Muller T, Rumpel E, Hradetzky S, Bollig F, Wegner H, et al. Non-muscle myosin IIA is required for the development of the zebrafish glomerulus. Kidney International. 2011; **80**:1055-1063. DOI: 10.1038/ki.2011.256

[62] Plaisier E, Alamowitch S, Gribouval O, Mougenot B, Gaudic A, et al. Autosomal-dominant familial hematuria with retinal arteriolar tortuosity and contractures: A novel syndrome. Kidney International. 2005;**67**:2354-2360. DOI: 10.1111/j.1523-1755.2005.00341.x

[63] Plaisier E, Chen Z, Gekeler F, Benhassine S, Dahan K, et al. Novel COL4A1 mutations associated with HANAC syndrome: A role for the triple helical CB3[IV] domain. American Journal of Medical Genetics. 2010;**152A**:2550-2555. DOI: 10.1002/ajmg.a.33659

[64] Longo I, Porcedda P, Mari F, Giachino D, Meloni I, et al. COL4A3/COL4A4 mutations: From familial hematuria to autosomal-dominant or recessive Alport syndrome. Kidney International. 2002;**61**(6):1947-1956. DOI: 10.1046/j.1523-1755.2002.00379.x

[65] Kashtan C. Renal transplantation in patients with Alport syndrome. Pediatric Transplantation. 2006;**10**:651-657. DOI: 10.1111/j.1399-3046.2006.00528.x

[66] Mojahedi M, Hekmat R, Ahmadnia H. Kidney transplantation in patients with Alport syndrome. Urology Journal. 2007;**4**:234-237 18270949

[67] Gumber M, Kute V, Goplani K, Vanikar A, Shah P, et al. Outcome of renal transplantation in Alport's syndrome: A single-center experience. Transplantation Proceedings. 2012;**44**:261-263. DOI: 10.1016/j.transproceed.2011.11.035

[68] Gross O, Beirowski B, Koepke M-L, Kuck J, Reiner M, et al. Preemptive ramipril therapy delays renal failure and reduces renal fibrosis in COL4A3-knockout mice with Alport syndrome. Kidney International. 2003;**63**:438-446. DOI: 10.1046/j.1523-1755.2003.00779.x

[69] Kashtan C, Ding J, Gregory M, Gross O, Heidet L, et al. Clinical practice recommendations for the treatment of Alport syndrome: A statement of the Alport syndrome research collaborative. Pediatric Nephrology. 2013;**28**(1):5-11. DOI: 10.1007/s00467-012-2138-4

[70] Gross O, Weber M. From the molecular genetics of Alport's syndrome to principles of organo-protection in chronic renal diseases. Medizinische Klinik. 2005;**100**:826-831. DOI: 10.1007/s00063-005-1114-1

[71] Gross O, Licht C, Anders H, Hoppe B, Beck B, et al. Early angiotensin-converting enzyme inhibition in Alport syndrome delays renal failure and improves life expectancy. Kidney International. 2012;**81**:494-501. DOI: 10.1038/ki.2011.407

[72] Gross O, Friede T, Hilgers R, Görlitz A, Gavénis K, et al. Safety and efficacy of the ACE-inhibitor ramipril in Alport syndrome: The double-blind, randomized, placebo-controlled, multicenter phase III EARLY PRO-TECT Alport trial in pediatric patients. ISRN Pediatrics. 2012;**2012**:436046. DOI: 10.5402/2012/436046

[73] Sayers R, Kalluri R, Rodgers K, Shield C, Meehan D, Cosgrove D. Role for transforming growth factor-β1 in Alport renal disease progression. Kidney International. 1999;**56**: 1662-1673

[74] Zeisberg M, Khurana M, Rao V, Cosgrove D, Rougier J-P, et al. Stage-specific action of matrix metalloproteinases influences progressive hereditary kidney disease. PLoS Medicine. 2006;**3**:e100. DOI: 10.1371/journal.pmed.0030100

[75] Koepke M, Weber M, Schulze-Lohoff E, Beirowski B, Segerer S, Gross O. Nephroprotective effect of the HMG CoA reductase inhibitor cerivastatin in a mouse model of progressive renal fibrosis in Alport syndrome. Nephrology, Dialysis, Transplantation. 2007;**22**:1062-1069. DOI: 10.1093/ndt/gfl810

[76] Ninichuk V, Gross O, Reichel C, Khandoga A, Pawar R, et al. Delayed chemokine receptor 1 blockade prolongs survival in collagen 4A3-deficient mice with Alport disease. JASN. 2005;**16**:977-985. DOI: 10.1681/ASN.2004100871

[77] Zeisberg M, Bottiglio C, Kumar N, Maeshima Y, Strutz F, et al. Bone morphogenic protein 7 inhibits progression of chronic renal fibrosis associated with two genetic mouse models. American Journal of Physiology. Renal Physiology. 2003;**285**:F1060-F1067. DOI: 10.1152/ajprenal.00191.2002

[78] Study of RG-012 in Male Subjects With Alport Syndrome (HERA). [Internet]. Available from: https://clinicaltrials.gov/ct2/show/NCT02855268 [Accessed: 2018.05.16]

[79] A Phase 2/3 Trial of the Efficacy and Safety of Bardoxolone Methyl in Patients With Alport Syndrome - CARDINAL (CARDINAL). [Internet]. Available from: https://clinicaltrials.gov/ct2/show/NCT03019185 [Accessed: 2018.05.16]

8

A Translational Metabonomic Assessment of Aristolochic Acid-Induced Nephropathies

Inès Jadot, Marilyn Duquesne,
Anne-Emilie Declèves, Nathalie Caron,
Jean-Marie Colet and Joëlle Nortier

Abstract

Aristolochic acid nephropathy (AAN) is a global term including any form of toxic interstitial nephropathy that is caused either by the ingestion of plants containing aristolochic acids (AA) as part of traditional phytotherapies or by the environmental contaminants in food. Originally, AAN was reported in Belgium in individuals having ingested slimming pills containing powdered root extracts of a Chinese herb, Aristolochia fangchi. However, it is estimated that exposure to AA affects thousands of people all over the world, particularly in the Balkans, Taiwan and China. Despite warnings from the Regulatory Agencies regarding the safety of products containing AA, many AAN cases remain frequently described worldwide. This chapter aims at giving a global picture of AAN through the descriptions of clinical cases and animal models, which were developed to better understand the mode of action of AA when inducing acute/chronic kidney diseases. Major advances in the translational research on biomarkers of AAN are reviewed, with an intended emphasis on the "omics" assessment of this nephrotoxicity.

Keywords: aristolochic acids, nephropathy, biomarkers, metabonomics, animal models

1. Introduction

The kidney plays a major role in the body homeostasis by regulating volume and composition of water fluids and by removing from blood waste products such as metabolites, drugs and xenobiotics. Due to these functions, the kidney is highly susceptible to toxic insults. During lifetime, the body is continuously exposed to numerous potentially toxic agents such as drugs

[1], chemicals and natural nephrotoxins [2]. Among these, herbal remedies and traditional phytotherapies constitute a major challenge. Indeed, traditional herbal remedies are considered harmless by the general population because they are from natural origin. Moreover, most patients using these natural products fail to inform their physicians of their use [2]. The following story demonstrates that the use of natural products, as all drugs, should be submitted to rigorous pharmacological and toxicological studies to determine their efficacy/safety. Some natural products have displayed therapeutic effects [3], whereas some others have been found to be highly toxic for the human body [4]. Among them, the toxicity of aristolochic acids (AA) has been extensively studied during the last decades. The term aristolochic acid nephropathy (AAN) includes any form of toxic interstitial nephropathy that is caused either by the ingestion of plants containing AA as part of traditional phytotherapies (formerly known as "Chinese herbs nephropathy") or by the environmental contaminants in food (Balkan endemic nephropathy, see below) [5]. AA are compounds found in plants from the genus Aristolochia, belonging to the plant family Aristolochiaceae. In addition to its nephrotoxic effects, AA exposure has also been frequently associated with the development of urothelial malignancies [6] and was classified as a human carcinogen class I by the World Health Organization (WHO) and the International Agency for Research on Cancer (IARC) in 2002 [7]. Since the identification of AAN in the early 1990s in Belgium [4], increasing cases of AA intoxications have been reported all over the world [8]. AAN incidence is particularly high in Asian countries because traditional medicines are very popular and the complexity of the pharmacopeia represents a high risk of AA intoxication due to some confusion between close species. In the Balkan areas, the chronic exposure to AA has been considered as the causative agent responsible for the so-called Balkan endemic nephropathy (BEN) that occurs following ingestion of food prepared with flour derived from contaminated grains [5, 9–14].

Despite warnings from the Food and Drug Administration (FDA), the European Medicines Agency (EMA) and IARC regarding the safety of products containing AA, AAN cases remain frequently described worldwide [5, 15, 16]. Moreover, given the fact that the nephrotoxic effect of AA is irreversible and that chronic kidney failure as well as carcinogenic effects may develop very slowly after the initial exposure, AAN and associated cancers are likely to become a major public health issue in the next few years [15, 16, 17].

This chapter aims at giving a global picture of AAN with an intended emphasis on the "omics" assessment of this nephrotoxicity, especially on the metabonomic investigation of urine samples. Indeed, it could represent a strategic tool allowing to identify early biomarkers following AA intoxication thereby providing an early detection of the toxicity and a rapid therapeutic intervention [18].

2. Clinical cases

Originally, AAN was reported in Belgium with more than 100 individuals having ingested slimming pills containing powdered root extracts of a Chinese herb, *Aristolochia fangchi* [4, 19]. A total of 75 patients have been treated in our Nephrology Department at Erasme Hospital. Among them, 50 out of 57 (F/M ratio 56/1) received a kidney transplant because of end-stage renal disease (ESRD); 21 presented with urothelial carcinoma of the upper tract (invasive in two cases) or the bladder (three cystectomies required), leading to five deaths. Four additional kidney recipients developed cancer of the digestive tract, one developed a brain lymphoma and 8 lethal cardiovascular or infectious complications. Among the seven patients still followed in 2018 for chronic kidney disease (CKD), a left nephroureterectomy had to be performed for pelvic carcinoma. Only one case of metastatic urothelial carcinoma was diagnosed without concomitant CKD [6]. The causal link with the intake of pills containing AA was demonstrated by the detection of DNA adducts specific to AA metabolites in renal tissue samples (see Section 3).

Although, initially, the Belgian cohort only included over 100 patients, it is estimated that exposure to AA affects 100,000 people in the Balkans (where the total number of patients with kidney disease amounts to approximately 25,000), 8,000,000 people in Taiwan and more than 100,000,000 in mainland China [20, 21]. In Asia, Aristolochia species is considered as an integral part of the herbology used in traditional Chinese medicine, Japanese Kampo and Ayurvedic medicine [8]. It is found within the same therapeutic family such as the Akebia, Asarum, Cocculus and Stephania plants. Referred by common names such as Mu Tong, Mokutsu and Fang Ji, they are used in a multitude of herbal mixtures for therapeutic use [22]. In the initial cohorts concerning iatrogenic nephropathy due to AA, most of the patients were described, exhibiting a rapid and progressive evolution toward CKD or ESRD [16]. A large series of patients described in China fixed the median rate of the degradation in glomerular filtration rate at ~3.5 ml/min/year [20]. The progression rate in environmental nephropathy due to AA is much slower, with the end-stage of renal failure occurring only after an evolution of 15–20 years [23].

3. Correlation between AA-DNA adducts, Aristolochic acid nephropathy and upper urinary tract carcinoma

Under normal physiological conditions, AA is bioactivated by the reduction of nitro compounds into "aristolactams," which tend to form covalent bonds with purine bases of DNA. The DNA adducts specific to aristolactams remain part of the body's cell structure for several years after the patients' initial exposure to AA. Consequently, their discovery in renal or cancerous tissues constitutes a biomarker, which may be related to a previous exposure to AA, which possibly occurred much earlier [24].

As mentioned earlier, 40–45% of end-stage AAN Belgian patients currently treated by dialysis or renal transplantation displayed multifocal high-grade transitional cell carcinomas, mainly in the upper urinary tract [6, 25]. As mentioned earlier, the detection of DNA adducts specific to AA metabolites (aristolactams) in nephroureterectomy pieces is still possible more than 10 years after exposure to AA [26]. The carcinogenic effect of AA can be explained by the fact that the DNA adducts formed in combination with aristolactams lead to a mutation of A: T →T: A in the tumor suppressor gene TP 53 [27]. This mutation has frequently been detected in the urothelial tumors of cases described in Taiwan and in the Balkans, whereas this mutation rarely occurs in tumors which are not related to the exposure to AA [28, 29]. This mutation is therefore considered as a complementary signature mutation for AA intoxication.

Besides the high prevalence of upper tract urothelial carcinoma, it must be underlined that cancers of the bladder appeared in female Belgian patients who had undergone transplants more than 15 years after exposure to AA had been stopped [30]. Frequent iatrogenic exposure to AA in Taiwan explains why this region has the world's highest level of urothelial cancers [31].

4. Experimental models of AA intoxication

In the 1980s, Mengs et al. had already pointed out AA toxicity and carcinogenicity in several experimental studies [32–34]. They developed diverse animal models using rats and mice of both sexes intoxicated with different doses of AA, during variable exposure times and using different routes of administration. They observed that oral or intravenous administration of high doses of AA was followed by death from acute renal failure within the next 15 days. The lethal dose 50 (LD_{50}) ranged from 56 to 203 mg/kg orally and 38 to 83 mg/kg intravenously, depending on species and gender [32]. Mengs reported that the kidneys were the most affected organs after intoxication confirming that they constitute AA main target [32].

Following the identification of AA as the agent responsible for AAN and BEN in 1993, various animal models were developed to study underlying mechanisms of AA nephrotoxicity. To do so, Cosyns et al. established a model of female New Zealand White rabbits injected intraperitoneally (i.p.) with 0.1 mg/kg of a mixture of AA (AAI: 44%; AAII: 56%), 5 days a week during 17–21 months [35]. The same authors reported the development of renal fibrosis and urothelial tumors in rabbits as it occurred in patients, therefore supporting the causal role of AA in the pathology.

Our group also developed different models of AAN. In 2002, Debelle et al. showed that daily subcutaneous injection of 10 mg/kg of AA mixture (AAI: 40%; AAII: 60%) in salt-depleted rats induced interstitial fibrosis and renal failure within 35 days [36]. In 2005, Lebeau et al. analyzed the time course of structural and functional impairments of the proximal tubule in a rat model of AAN using the same protocol [37]. A biphasic evolution of renal dysfunction and morphological alterations was described. First, a phase of acute kidney injury (AKI) was characterized with structural abnormalities occurring within the first 3 days as attested by necrosis of proximal tubular epithelial cells (PTEC). Dysfunction of proximal tubule was also highlighted by an increase of biochemical parameters such as tubular proteinuria, N-acetyl-β-D-glucosaminidase (NAG), α-glutathione S-transferase (α-GST), leucine aminopeptidase (LAP) and neutral endopeptidase (NEP) enzymuria. At day 35 of the protocol, a second phase was identified, mainly associated to morphological alterations along with the presence of severe tubular atrophy in an interstitial fibrotic environment. Moreover, tubular proteinuria, NAG, α-GST, LAP and NEP enzymuria were further enhanced at this timepoint characterizing the later phase of chronic kidney injury.

Regarding mice models, it has been shown that mice from different strains displayed variable susceptibility to AA treatment. In this regard, Sato et al. published a study in which they compared three strains of inbred mice, BALB/c, C3H/He and C57BL/6 that received 2.5 mg/kg of AA (AAI: 55%; AAII: 45%) or AA sodium salt daily by i.p. injection or oral administration,

5 days a week for 2 weeks [38]. Characteristic tubulointerstitial lesions as well as parameters of renal dysfunction were observed in both strains intoxicated with AA. However, the susceptibility to AA differed between the three strains tested. The authors postulated that these differences might reflect diversity in AA metabolism and/or in the mechanisms of detoxification. Indeed, genetic polymorphisms have been identified as a major factor affecting the expression level and/or activity of enzymes involved in AA metabolism. The variations observed between the different strains could therefore be linked to such polymorphisms.

More recently, we also confirmed the biphasic evolution in a mouse model of AAN (**Figure 1**). C57Bl/6 J male mice were daily i.p. injected with a solution of AAI (3.5 mg/kg) for 4 days and then sacrificed at 5, 10 or 20 days after the first day of injection [15, 39]. The acute phase was identified at day 5 with necrosis of PTEC while at day 20, cystic tubules and tubulointerstitial fibrosis was observed characterizing the features of a chronic phase. This transition from AKI to CKD has an important significance clinically. Indeed, it has been shown that patients surviving an episode of AKI present a significant risk of progression to CKD [40–42]. However, the mechanisms by which AKI might initiate the onset of CKD have not been fully described. Therefore, a better understanding of the pathological mechanisms of AAN along with the identification of early biomarkers could lead to therapeutic strategies to treat AKI or impede progression to CKD. Along these lines, animal models of AAN could be considered as a useful tool providing important insight on the underlying mechanisms of AKI-to-CKD transition. In this regard, we recently demonstrated that renal nitric oxide (NO) bioavailability was significantly reduced during the AKI-to-CKD transition in our AAN model while L-Arginine supplementation appeared beneficial [39]. Indeed, L-Arg treatment restored renal NO bioavailability and reduced the severity of tubular necrosis, inflammation and fibrosis

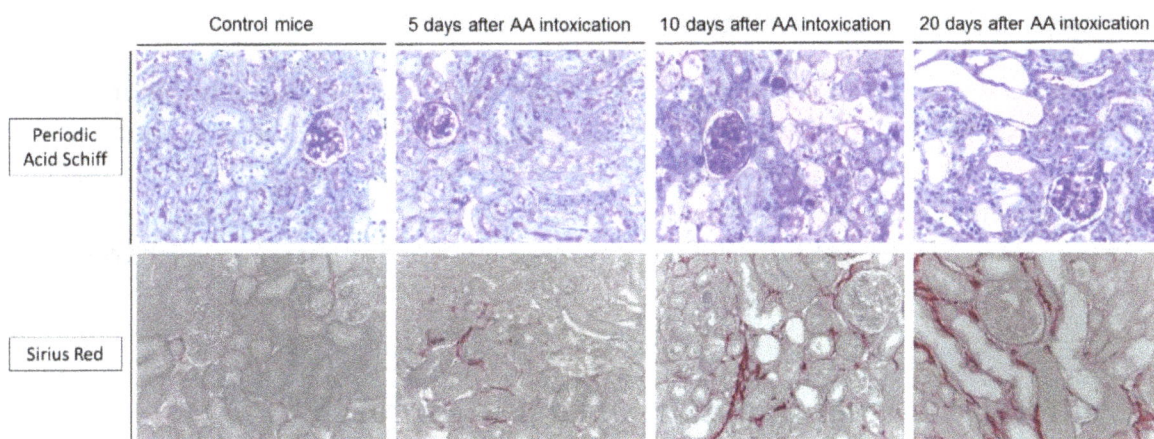

Figure 1. Renal histology of AA-induced tissue injury. A–D. Representative photomicrographs (×400 magnification) illustrating renal tissue injury with periodic acid-Schiff staining in Ctl (A), 5 days after AA intoxication (B), 10 days after AA intoxication (C) and 20 days after AA intoxication (D). Zones of necrotic proximal tubular epithelial cells are observed in AA intoxication at day 5, 10 and 20 after AA (B-D). Moreover, cystic tubules and proteinuria (*) are visible in mice treated with AA at day 10 and 20. E–H. representative photomicrographs (×400 magnification) illustrating collagen deposit with Sirius red staining in Ctl (E), 5 days after AA intoxication (F), 10 days after AA intoxication (G) and 20 days after AA intoxication (H). Deposition of collagen I and III are observed in the interstitium of renal parenchyma in AA-treated mice at day 5 (D). Collagen deposition are even enhanced from day 10 to day 20 (G–H). Abbreviations: G, glomerulus; NT, necrotic tubule; CT: cystic tubules and PT, proximal tubule.

AA-intoxicated mice. We concluded that reduced NO bioavailability contributes to the pathological processes in AAN but also that L-Arg could represent a potential therapeutic tool to decrease the severity of acute-to-chronic transition.

5. Conventional biomarkers

In most AAN cases, renal failure was discovered by routine blood testing [43]. Typically, moderate hypertension developed with increased serum creatinine and severe anemia [8, 44]. Proteinuria from tubular origin was confirmed with elevated urinary excretion of five low molecular weight proteins (β2-microglobulin, cystatin C, Clara cell protein, retinal-binding protein and α1-microglobulin) [45]. Levels of urinary neutral endopeptidase (NEP), a 94 kDa ectoenzyme of the proximal tubule brush border, constitute a reliable indicator of the severity of renal disease. Indeed, it has been shown to reflect the proportion of brush borders remaining intact at the apical side of proximal tubules. Urinary NEP was significantly decreased in patient with moderate renal failure and almost undetectable in those with ESRD, indicating the loss of the proximal tubule integrity [46]. A hallmark of the Belgian cohort of AAN cases is the rapid progression to an ESRD in nearly 70% of intoxicated patients [44]. The combination of rapidly progressive interstitial renal fibrosis with urothelial malignancy strongly suggests the diagnostic of AAN. Since 2015, a consensus regarding the definition of diagnostic criteria has been established [16]. AAN will be diagnosed in any individual who suffers from renal failure in combination with at least two of the following three criteria: (1) a renal histology highlighting interstitial fibrosis distributed along a corticomedullary gradient; (2) a history of herbal products consumption with the demonstration of the presence of AA and (3) the identification of AA-DNA adducts or the specific A:T $\rightarrow$ T:A transversion in the tumor suppressor gene TP 53 in a kidney tissue sample or in a urothelial tumor.

Until now, no serum or urinary biomarker has been identified for clinical utility in the diagnosis of AAN or BEN [16]. Although mechanistically informative, the conventional markers described in the previous paragraph display a lack of sensitivity. When abnormal levels of those markers are noticed, irreversible damages were already set up. In this regard, the 'omics' approach could constitute a strategic tool to identify early markers which could allow an early therapeutic intervention [18].

6. Nephrotoxicity assessment by the 'omics' approach

The biomarkers conventionally used in toxicology are particularly useful to detect or to follow the evolution of a very specific effect usually identified in advance. On the other hand, significant variations in the levels of such biomarkers are often too late since they only appear once severe or worse irreversible damages are already developed. Moreover, they are not appropriate to identify unknown or unexpected effects or to appreciate responses that result from several effects occurring simultaneously in various cell types, organs or systems.

Toxicogenomics is a more recent discipline that broadly studies changes in genes (genomics), RNA (transcriptomics), proteins (proteomics) and metabolites (metabol(n)omics) in a whole living organism exposed to a xenobiotic substance causing subsequent adverse health effects [47]. The main goal in toxicogenomics is to obtain a global and integrated view of the molecular and cellular mechanisms underlying a toxic response. It is crucial to distinguish changes in basal expression, for example due to stress, from both adaptive and toxic responses. In addition, according to the principle of molecular homology, it is likely that substances sharing similar chemical structures will display close mode of toxic action by altering the same set of genes, proteins and metabolites. Therefore, reference databases can be built that contain characteristic expression profiles of reference toxicants [48]. The comparison of the expression profile induced by a tested molecule with the database allows a fine classification. From the properties of the identified class, the toxic behavior of the test substance can be predicted. Finally, thanks to the development of 'high-throughput' analytical techniques, the expression of thousands of genes at the level of RNA or proteins can be simultaneously measured in an organ/tissue subjected to the effect of a toxic substance. In parallel, changes in the metabolic composition of biofluids and biopsies can be assessed over time. These global measurements facilitate not only the observation of the effects of a molecule on the targeted tissues (on-target), but also of the harmful effects on non-targeted tissues (off-target) [49].

In a recent review, conventional and toxicogenomics methods were compared to evaluate their potential to predict nephrotoxicity, genotoxicity and teratogenicity of traditional remedies [50]. Toxicogenomics methods present the main advantage to allow a quick and simultaneous acquisition of multiple markers which can be next identified and related to cellular processes targeted by the tested compound. Focusing on the nephrotoxicity assessment, these new approaches could identify a set of proteins and metabolites which might be promising biomarkers indicative of very early cellular changes. Compared to conventional markers such as plasma creatinine and BUN, the "omics" indicators are more sensitive and more specific. On the protein side, Clusterin, Cystatin-C, and N-Gal/lipolcalin-2, among others, are now considered as excellent candidates to detect acute or chronic tubulotoxicity [51, 52] to such an extent that they have been accepted by regulatory agencies (FDA and EMA) for the detection of acute kidney injury in preclinical risk assessment. On the metabolite side, since the COMET (Consortium for Metabonomic Toxicology) project that evaluated the benefit of metabonomics in the prediction of potential drug adverse effect [48], numerous nonclinical and clinical studies have reported the usefulness of urine metabolic markers to predict acute and chronic renal injuries. In rats, variations in plasma 3-methylhistidine (3-MH) and 3-indoxyl sulfate (3-IS) are now recognized as early predictors of a decline in glomerular filtration due to acute renal failure, while the combination of simultaneous changes in urine glucose, methylamines, hippurate and certain amino acids is associated with proximal tubule damages [53].

Of course, those new approaches in systems biology are far from being validated. Nevertheless, in association with *in vivo* models, they are already useful to mechanistically assess the nephrotoxicity of xenobiotics. Most importantly, many recent studies highlight their unique potential for translational research from benchside to bedside, especially for the diagnosis and follow up of AKI [54].

Both genomic and transcriptomic approaches have already been applied to investigate the cellular mechanisms of AA toxicity and tentatively reveal fingerprints of AA exposure. Human exome sequencing of urothelial carcinoma of the upper urinary tract from individuals chronically exposed to AA revealed characteristic and unusual somatic mutations predominantly located on the non-transcribed strand [55]. This AA-related mutational fingerprint was essentially found in oncogenes and tumor suppressor genes. Using a molecular epidemiologic approach based on genome sequencing, the genome-wide mutational signature for AA was also detected in liver and kidney cancers in targeted Taiwanese and Chinese populations [56, 57]. Exposure to AA in various animal species and in humans is detected by the presence of aristolactam-DNA adducts, with excellent results obtained on renal specimens by ultra-performance liquid chromatography-electrospray ionization/multistage mass spectrometry (UPLC-ESI/MSn) [58]. Such DNA adducts represent the direct evidence of tissue exposure to AA, and according to these authors, they can serve as endpoints for cross-species extrapolation of toxicity data and human risk assessment.

Proteomic analyses of urinary, plasma and renal tissue resulted in differential expression of several cytoskeletal, developmental and inflammatory kidney proteins, in both AA-exposed and control mice [59]. Using fluorogenic derivatization followed by high-performance liquid chromatography analysis and liquid chromatography tandem mass spectrometry with a MASCOT database searching system, two altered proteins, thrombospondin type 1 and a G protein-coupled receptor, were identified as discriminating mice chronically exposed to AA [60]. A proteomic signature of AA-exposure was also identified in rat kidney: upregulated proteins included ornithine aminotransferase, sorbitol dehydrogenase, actin, aspartoacylase, 3-hydroxyisobutyrate dehydrogenase and peroxiredoxin-1, while ATP synthase subunit β, glutamate dehydrogenase 1, regucalcin, glutamate-cysteine ligase regulatory subunit, dihydropteridine reductase, hydroxyacyl-coenzyme A dehydrogenase, voltage-dependent anion-selective channel protein 1, prohibitin, and adenylate kinase isoenzyme 4 were all downregulated [61]. Interestingly, some of those proteins presented obvious biological and medical significance.

From the metabol(n)omics side, several studies were conducted either in experimental animal models or in patients. For example, a GC-MS-based metabolomic study was performed to analyze urinary metabolites in AA-exposed rats over time [62]. Among all metabolic alterations, eight metabolites were selected as potential metabolic biomarkers including methylsuccinic acid, nicotinamide, 3-hydroxyphenylacetic acid, citric acid, creatinine, uric acid, glycolic acid and gluconic acid. Four of them were considered as "early indicator" (methylsuccinic acid, citric acid, creatinine and 3-hydroxyphenylacetic acid), while the others were defined as "late metabolic biomarker." According to the authors, the metabolomics markers were more sensitive than conventional biomarkers of renal injury. Using a UPLC/QTOF-HDMS analysis, a bench of lipids molecules including cholic and chenodeoxycholic acid were identified as excellent biomarkers to evaluate the progression from early to advanced AAN. Also, indoxyl sulfate, uric acid and creatinine were considered as good markers in severe cases of AAN. Interestingly, they were also reversible under treatments both in AAN rats and in CKD patients [63]. Using a ^{1}H-NMR-based approach, we compared the urine metabonomic profiles of rats exposed to either AAI, AAII, or the mixture. Metabolic alterations indicating a proximal tubule injury were observed in all treated groups. These dose-dependent effects already noticed at early stages were morphologically confirmed at later

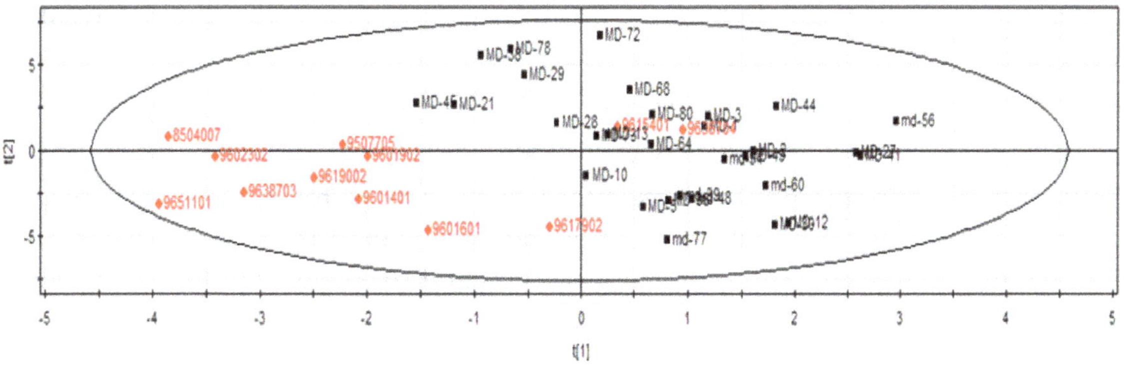

Figure 2. Scores plot comparing the ¹HNMR spectra of urine samples from diseased Balkan women in red with the urine samples collected from healthy Belgian women, in black. PLS-DA model.

time points. Renal damages were more pronounced with the mixture or AAII alone than AAI alone [18].

¹H NMR-based metabolomics was also applied to urine samples collected from BEN-diagnosed people treated by hemodialysis, in Romania and Bulgaria [64]. While samples from healthy volunteers from both countries coincided in the PCA scores plot, Bulgarian and Romanian BEN-suffering patients not only deviated from controls but also from each other. This study also suggested that metabonomic assessment could be predictive of impending morbidity before conventional criteria can diagnose BEN. Similar metabonomic approach was also applied to surplus of urine samples collected from Belgian women (acutely and mistakenly exposed to AA through diet pills) and Croatian patients (chronically exposed to AA through contaminated food) [65] (**Figure 2**). Interestingly, a clear discrimination of the Belgian patients from healthy volunteers was shown, and urine samples collected from individuals living in Croatian endemic regions as compared to Croatian inhabitants from non-endemic villages tended to separate from each other. Finally, both Belgian and Croatian patients displayed close urine metabolic profiles, suggesting a common etiology of both diseases.

In conclusion, the methods in toxicogenomics have already brought water to the mill of researches on nephropathies induced by AA. Thus, aristolactam-DNA adducts specific to the AA exposure were revealed by genomic methods. For their part, proteomic and metabolomic approaches have identified very early and specific biomarkers of tubular renal damage associated with exposure to AA. These same markers have also opened new mechanistic tracks on the toxic modes of action of AA at the molecular and cellular levels.

7. Conclusions

"AAN" is a global designation for any toxic interstitial nephropathy consecutive to the exposure to aristolochic acids. Although the development of accurate experimental models and the validation of robust biomarkers these last decades have allowed a better mechanistic understanding of the mode of action of those natural substances, we are still facing many challenges. In particular, the need for early and more predictive indicators of AAN in both animal models and in clinics is urgent. Also, unveiling the role of altered renal hemodynamics in the pathogenesis as well as the molecular and cellular events leading from an acute to a chronic kidney disease in patients is essential. To this respect, the omics technologies have already brought new pieces to the puzzle. Specifically, metabonomic applied to urine samples collected from AA-exposed animals or AAN patients stands out as a very promising approach.

More philosophically, the history of AAN reminds us that natural products are not without risk. The easy and uncontrolled access to such substances, for instance from suspicious sources on the Web, increases the risk of renewing this sad experience. A review of the most recent literature in the field of traditional medicines and remedies reinforces our belief that they should be subject to the same safety assessments as drugs, and that omic methods should be included at different steps of the assessment process.

Conflict of interest

Authors declare no conflict of interest.

Author details

Inès Jadot[1], Marilyn Duquesne[2], Anne-Emilie Declèves[2], Nathalie Caron[1], Jean-Marie Colet[2]* and Joëlle Nortier[3]

*Address all correspondence to: joelle.nortier@erasme.ulb.ac.be

1 University of Namur, Namur, Belgium

2 University of Mons, Mons, Belgium

3 Free University of Brussels, Brussels, Belgium

References

[1] Tiong HY, Huang P, Xiong S, et al. Drug-induced nephrotoxicity: Clinical impact and preclinical in vitro models. Molecular Pharmaceutics. 2014;**11**:1933-1948. DOI: 10.1021/mp400720w

[2] Nauffal M, Gabardi S. Nephrotoxicity of natural products. Blood Purification. 2016;**41**:123-129. DOI: 10.1159/000441268

[3] Zhong Y, Deng Y, Chen Y, et al. Therapeutic use of traditional Chinese herbal medications for chronic kidney diseases. Kidney International. 2013;**84**:1108-1118. DOI: 10.1038/ki.2013.276

[4] Vanherweghem J-L, Depierreux MF, Tielemans C, et al. Rapidly progressive interstitial renal fibrosis in young women: Association with slimming regimen including Chinese herbs. Lancet. 1993;**341**:387-391. DOI: 10.1186/1752-1947-4-409

[5] De Broe ME. Chinese herbs nephropathy and Balkan endemic nephropathy: Toward a single entity, aristolochic acid nephropathy. Kidney International. 2012;**81**:513-515. DOI: 10.1038/ki.2011.428

[6] Nortier JL, Muniz Martinez M-C, Schmeiser HH, et al. Urothelial carcinoma associated with the use of a Chinese herb. The New England Journal of Medicine. 2000;**342**:1686-1692. DOI: 10.1056/NEJM200006083422301

[7] National Toxicology Program. Aristolochic Acids. Rep. Carcinog; 2008

[8] Debelle F, Vanherweghem J-L, Nortier JL. Aristolochic acid nephropathy: A worldwide problem. Kidney International. 2008;**74**:158-169. DOI: 10.1038/ki.2008.129

[9] Cosyns J-P, Jadoul M, Squifflet J-P, et al. Chinese herbs nephropathy : A clue to Balkan endemic nephropathy ? Kidney International. 1994;**45**:1680-1688. DOI: 10.1038/ki.1994.220

[10] Arlt VM, Ferluga D, Stiborová M, et al. Is aristolochic acid a risk factor for Balkan endemic nephropathy-associated urothelial cancer? International Journal of Cancer. 2002;**101**:500-502. DOI: 10.1002/ijc.10602

[11] Arlt VM, Alunni-Perret V, Quatrehomme G, et al. Aristolochic acid (AA)-DNA adduct as marker of AA exposure and risk factor for AA nephropathy-associated cancer. International Journal of Cancer. 2004;**111**:977-980. DOI: 10.1002/ijc.20316

[12] Samardzic J, Hasukic S. Upper urinary tract urothelial cancer in croatian and bosnian endemic nephropathy regions. Medieval Archaeology. 2017;**71**:430. DOI: 10.5455/medarh.2017.71.430-433

[13] Chan W, Pavlovic N. Quantitation of aristolochic acids in corn, wheat grain, and soil samples collected in Serbia: Identifying a novel exposure pathway in the etiology of balkan endemic nephropathy. Journal of Agricultural and Food Chemistry. 2016;**64**(29):5928-5934. DOI: 10.1021/acs.jafc.6b02203

[14] Gruia AT, Oprean C, Ivan A, et al. Balkan endemic nephropathy and aristolochic acid I: An investigation into the role of soil and soil organic matter contamination, as a potential natural exposure pathway. Environmental Geochemistry and Health. 2017;**39**:1-12. DOI: 10.1007/s10653-017-0065-9

[15] Jadot I, Declèves A-E, Nortier JL, et al. An integrated view of aristolochic acid nephropathy: Update of the literature. International Journal of Molecular Sciences. 2017;**18**:1-23. DOI: 10.3390/ijms18020297

[16] Gökmen MR, Cosyns JP, Arlt VM, et al. The epidemiology, diagnosis, and management of aristolochic acid nephropathy: A narrative review. Annals of Internal Medicine. 2013;**158**:469-477. DOI: 10.7326/0003-4819-158-6-201303190-00006

[17] Bunel V, Souard F, Antoine MH, Stevigny C, Nortier JL. Nephrotoxicity of natural products: Aristolochic acid and fungal toxins. In: McQueen CA, editor. Comprehensive Toxicology. 3rd ed. Vol. 14. Oxford Elsevier Ltd; 2018. pp. 340-379. DOI: 10.1016/B978-0-12-801238-3.64093-X

[18] Duquesne M, Declèves AE, De Prez E, et al. Interest of metabonomic approach in environmental nephrotoxicants: Application to aristolochic acid exposure. Food and Chemical Toxicology. 2017;**108**:19-29. DOI: 10.1016/j.fct.2017.07.015

[19] Vanhaelen M, Vanhaelen-Fastre R, But P, Vanherweghem JL. Identification of aristolochic acid in Chinese herbs. Lancet. 1994;**343**:174. DOI: 10.1016/S0140-6736(94)90964-4

[20] Yang L, Su T, Li XM, et al. Aristolochic acid nephropathy: Variation in presentation and prognosis. Nephrology, Dialysis, Transplantation. 2012;**27**:292-298. DOI: 10.1093/ndt/gfr291

[21] Hsieh SC, Lin IH, Tseng WL, et al. Prescription profile of potentially aristolochic acid containing Chinese herbal products: An analysis of national health insurance data in Taiwan between 1997 and 2003. Chinese Medicine. 2008;**3**:13. DOI: 10.1186/1749-8546-3-13

[22] Heinrich M, Chan J, Wanke S, et al. Local uses of Aristolochia species and content of nephrotoxic aristolochic acid 1 and 2-a global assessment based on bibliographic sources. Journal of Ethnopharmacology. 2009;**125**:108-144. DOI: 10.1016/j.jep.2009.05.028

[23] Pavlovic NM. Balkan endemic nephropathy - current status and future perspectives. Clinical Kidney Journal. 2013;**6**:257-265. DOI: 10.1093/ckj/sft049

[24] Arlt VM, Stiborova M, Schmeiser HH. Aristolochic acid as a probable human cancer hazard in herbal remedies: A review. Mutagenesis. 2002;**17**:265-277. DOI: 10.1093/mutage/17.4.265

[25] Cosyns JP, Jadoul M, Squifflet JP, et al. Urothelial lesions in Chinese-herb nephropathy. American Journal of Kidney Diseases. 1999;**33**:1011-1017. DOI: 10.1016/S0272-6386(99)70136-8

[26] Schmeiser HH, Nortier JL, Singh R, et al. Exceptionally long-term persistence of DNA adducts formed by carcinogenic aristolochic acid I in renal tissue from patients with aristolochic acid nephropathy. International Journal of Cancer. 2014;**135**:502-507. DOI: 10.1002/ijc.28681

[27] Stiborova M, Arlt VM, Schmeiser HH. DNA adducts formed by aristolochic acid are unique biomarkers of exposure and explain the initiation phase of upper urothelial cancer. International Journal of Molecular Sciences. 2017;**18**:E2144. DOI: 10.3390/ijms18102144

[28] Chen CH, Dickman KG, Huang CY, et al. Aristolochic acid-induced upper tract urothelial carcinoma in Taiwan: Clinical characteristics and outcomes. International Journal of Cancer. 2013;**133**:14-20. DOI: 0.1002/ijc.28013

[29] Jelaković B, Karanović S, Vuković-Lela I, et al. Aristolactam-DNA adducts are a biomarker of environmental exposure to aristolochic acid. Kidney International. 2012;**81**:559-567. DOI: 10.1038/ki.2011.371

[30] Lemy A, Wissing KM, Rorive S, et al. Late onset of bladder urothelial carcinoma after kidney transplantation for end-stage aristolochic acid nephropathy: A case series with 15-year follow-up. American Journal of Kidney Diseases. 2008;**51**:471-477. DOI: 10.1053/j.ajkd.2007.11.015

[31] Grollman AP. Aristolochic acid nephropathy: Harbinger of a global iatrogenic disease. Environmental and Molecular Mutagenesis. 2013;**54**:1-7. DOI: 10.1002/em.21756

[32] Mengs U. Acute toxicity of aristolochic acid in rodents. Archives of Toxicology. 1987; **59**:328-331. DOI: 10.1007/BF00295084

[33] Mengs U. Tumor induction in mice following exposure to aristolochic acid. Archives of Toxicology. 1988;**61**:504-505. DOI: 10.1007/BF00293699

[34] Mengs U, Lang W, Poch J-A. The carcinogenic action of aristolochic acid in rats. Archives of Toxicology. 1982;**51**:107-119. DOI: 10.1007/BF00302751

[35] Cosyns J-P, Dehoux JP, Guiot Y, et al. Chronic aristolochic acid toxicity in rabbits: A model of Chinese herbs nephropathy? Kidney International. 2001;**59**:2164-2173. DOI: 10.1046/j.1523-1755.2001.0590062164.x

[36] Debelle F, Nortier J, De Prez E, Garbar C, Vienne A, Salmon I, Deschodt-Lanckman M, Vanherwehem J-L. Aristolochic Acids Induce Chronic Renal Failure with Interstitial Fibrosis in Salt-Depleted Rats. Journal of the American Society of Nephrology. 2002; **13**:431-436. DOI: 1046-6673/1302-0431

[37] Lobeau C, Debelle F, Arlt VM, et al. Early proximal tubule injury in experimental aristolochic acid nephropathy: Functional and histological studies. Nephrology, Dialysis, Transplantation. 2005;**20**:2321-2332. DOI: 10.1093/ndt/gfi042

[38] Sato N, Takahashi D, Chen SM, Tsuchiya R, Mukoyama T, Yamagata S, Ogawa M, Yoshida M, Kondo S, Satoh N, Ueda S. Acute nephrotoxicity of aristolochic acids in mice. The Journal of Pharmacy and Pharmacology. 2004;**56**(2):221-229. DOI: 10.1211/0022357023051

[39] Jadot I, Colombaro V, Martin B, et al. Restored nitric oxide bioavailability reduces the severity of acute-to-chronic transition in a mouse model of aristolochic acid nephropathy. PLoS One. 2017;**12**:1-19. DOI: 10.1371/journal. pone.0183604

[40] Zuk A, Bonventre JV. Acute Kidney Injury. Annual Review of Medicine. 2016;**67**:293-307. DOI: 10.1016/B978-1-4557-4555-5.00110-2

[41] Chawla LS, Amdur RL, Amodeo S, et al. The severity of acute kidney injury predicts progression to chronic kidney disease. Kidney International. 2011;**79**:1361-1369. DOI: 10.1038/ki.2011.42

[42] Chawla LS, Eggers PW, Star RA, et al. Acute kidney injury and chronic kidney disease as interconnected syndromes. The New England Journal of Medicine. 2014;**371**:58-66. DOI: 10.1056/NEJMra1214243

[43] Nortier JL, Pozdzik A, Roumeguere T, et al. Néphropathie aux acides aristolochiques (« néphropathie aux herbes chinoises »). Néphrologie & Thérapeutique. 2015;**11**:574-588. DOI: 10.1016/j.nephro.2015.10.001

[44] Reginster F, Jadoul M, Van Ypersele De Strihou C. Chinese herbs nephropathy presentation, natural history and fate after transplantation. Nephrology, Dialysis, Transplantation. 1997;**12**:81-86. DOI: 10.1093/ndt/12.1.81

[45] Kabanda A, Jadoul M, Lauwerys R, et al. Low molecular weight proteinuria in Chinese herbs nephropathy. Kidney International. 1995;**48**:1571-1576. DOI: 10.1038/ki.1995.449

[46] Nortier JL, Deschodt-Lanckman M, Simon S, et al. Proximal tubular injury in Chinese herbs nephropathy: Monitoring by neutral endopeptidase enzymuria. Kidney International. 1997;**51**:288-293. DOI: 10.1038/ki.1997.35

[47] Buesen R, Chorley BN, Silva Lima B, et al. Applying 'omics technologies in chemicals risk assessment: Report of an ECETOC workshop. Regulatory Toxicology and Pharmacology. 2017;**91**(S1):S3-S13. DOI: 10.1016/j.yrtph.2017.09.002

[48] Lindon JC, Keun HC, Ebbels TM, Pearce JM, Holmes E, Nicholson JK. The Consortium for Metabonomic Toxicology (COMET): Aims, activities and achievements. Pharmacogenomics. 2005;**6**(7):691-699. DOI: 10.2217/14622416.6.7.691

[49] Colet JM. Metabonomics in the preclinical and environmental toxicity field. Drug Discovery Today: Technologies. 2015;**13**:3-10. DOI: 10.1016/j.ddtec.2015.01.002

[50] Ouedraogo M, Baudoux T, Stévigny C, Nortier J, Colet JM, Efferth T, Qu F, Zhou J, Chan K, Shaw D, Pelkonen O, Duez P. Review of current and "omics" methods for assessing the toxicity (genotoxicity, teratogenicity and nephrotoxicity) of herbal medicines and mushrooms. Journal of Ethnopharmacology. 2012;**140**(3):492-512. DOI: 10.1016/j.jep.2012.01.059

[51] Hoffmann D, Fuchs TC, Henzler T, Matheis KA, Herget T, Dekant W, Hewitt P, Mally A. Evaluation of a urinary kidney biomarker panel in rat models of acute and subchronic nephrotoxicity. Toxicology. 2010;**277**(1-3):49-58. DOI: 10.1016/j.tox.2010.08.013

[52] Marrer E, Dieterle F. Impact of biomarker development on drug safety assessment. Toxicology and Applied Pharmacology. 2010;**243**(2):167-179. DOI: 10.1016/j.taap.2009.12.015

[53] Uehara T, Horinouchi A, Morikawa Y, Tonomura Y, Minami K, Ono A, Yamate J, Yamada H, Ohno Y, Urushidani T. Identification of metabolomic biomarkers for drug-induced acute kidney injury in rats. Journal of Applied Toxicology. 2014;**34**(10):1087-1095. DOI: 10.1002/jat.2933

[54] Marx D, Metzger J, Pejchinovski M, RB4 G, Frantzi M, Latosinska A, Belczacka I, Heinzmann SS, Husi H, Zoidakis J, Klingele M, Herget-Rosenthal S. Proteomics and Metabolomics for AKI Diagnosis. Seminars in Nephrology. 2018;**38**(1):63-87. DOI: 10.1016/j.semnephrol.2017.09.007

[55] Hoang ML, Chen CH, Sidorenko VS, He J, Dickman KG, Yun BH, Moriya M, Niknafs N, Douville C, Karchin R, Turesky RJ, Pu YS, Vogelstein B, Papadopoulos N, Grollman AP, Kinzler KW, Rosenquist TA. Mutational signature of aristolochic acid exposure as revealed by whole-exome sequencing. Science Translational Medicine. 2013;**5**(197):197. DOI: 10.1126/scitranslmed.3006200

[56] Rosenquist TA, Grollman AP. Mutational signature of aristolochic acid: Clue to the recognition of a global disease. DNA Repair (Amst). 2016;**44**:205-211. DOI: 10.1016/j.dnarep.2016.05.027

[57] Ng AWT, Poon SL, Huang MN, Lim JQ, Boot A, Yu W, Suzuki Y, Thangaraju S, Ng CCY, Tan P, Pang ST, Huang HY, Yu MC, Lee PH, Hsieh SY, Chang AY, Teh BT, Rozen SG. Aristolochic acids and their derivatives are widely implicated in liver cancers in Taiwan and throughout Asia. Science Translational Medicine. 2017;**9**(412). DOI: 10.1126/scitranslmed.aan6446

[58] Yun BH, Sidorenko VS, Rosenquist TA, Dickman KG, Grollman AP, Turesky RJ. New approaches for biomonitoring exposure to the human carcinogen aristolochic acid. Toxicology Research (Camb). 2015;**4**(4):763-776. DOI: 10.1039/C5TX00052A

[59] Rucevic M, Rosenquist T, Breen L, Cao L, Clifton J, Hixson D, Josic D. Proteome alterations in response to aristolochic acids in experimental animal model. Journal of Proteomics. 2012;**76**:79-90. DOI: 10.1016/j.jprot.2012.06.026

[60] Lin CE, Chang WS, Lee JA, Chang TY, Huang YS, Hirasaki Y, Chen HS, Imai K, Chen SM. Proteomics analysis of altered proteins in kidney of mice with aristolochic acid nephropathy using the fluorogenic derivatization-liquid chromatography-tandem mass spectrometry method. Biomedical Chromatography. 2018;**32**(3):e-4127. DOI: 10.1002/bmc.4127

[61] Wu HZ, Guo L, Mak YF, Liu N, Poon WT, Chan YW, Cai Z. Proteomics investigation on aristolochic acid nephropathy: A case study on rat kidney tissues. Analytical and Bioanalytical Chemistry. 2011;**399**(10):3431-3439. DOI: 10.1007/s00216-010-4463-4

[62] Hu X, Shen J, Pu X, Zheng N, Deng Z, Zhang Z, Li H. Urinary time- or dose-dependent metabolic biomarkers of aristolochic acid-induced nephrotoxicity in rats. Toxicological Sciences. 2017;**156**(1):123-132. DOI: 10.1093/toxsci/kfw244

[63] Hua C, Gang C, Dan-Qian C, Ming W, Nosratola DV, Zhi-Hao Z, Jia-Rong M, Xu B, Ying-Yong Z. Metabolomics insights into activated redox signaling and lipid metabolism dysfunction in chronic kidney disease progression. Redox Biology. 2016;**10**:168-178. DOI: 10.1016/j.redox.2016.09.014

[64] Mantle P, Modalca M, Nicholls A, Tatu C, Tatu D, Toncheva D. Comparative (1)H NMR metabolomic urinalysis of people diagnosed with Balkan endemic nephropathy, and healthy subjects, in Romania and Bulgaria: A pilot study. Toxins (Basel). 2011;**3**(7):815-833. DOI: 10.3390/toxins3070815

[65] Duquesne M, Goossens C, Dika Ž, Conotte R, Nortier J, Jelaković B, Colet JM. Metabonomics: On the road to detect diagnostic biomarkers in endemic (Balkan) nephropathy. Evaluation in a retrospective pilot project. Journal of Cancer Science and Therapy. 2013;**S18**:2012. DOI: 10.4172/1948-5956.S18-002

Permissions

All chapters in this book were first published in AN, by InTech Open; hereby published with permission under the Creative Commons Attribution License or equivalent. Every chapter published in this book has been scrutinized by our experts. Their significance has been extensively debated. The topics covered herein carry significant findings which will fuel the growth of the discipline. They may even be implemented as practical applications or may be referred to as a beginning point for another development.

The contributors of this book come from diverse backgrounds, making this book a truly international effort. This book will bring forth new frontiers with its revolutionizing research information and detailed analysis of the nascent developments around the world.

We would like to thank all the contributing authors for lending their expertise to make the book truly unique. They have played a crucial role in the development of this book. Without their invaluable contributions this book wouldn't have been possible. They have made vital efforts to compile up to date information on the varied aspects of this subject to make this book a valuable addition to the collection of many professionals and students.

This book was conceptualized with the vision of imparting up-to-date information and advanced data in this field. To ensure the same, a matchless editorial board was set up. Every individual on the board went through rigorous rounds of assessment to prove their worth. After which they invested a large part of their time researching and compiling the most relevant data for our readers.

The editorial board has been involved in producing this book since its inception. They have spent rigorous hours researching and exploring the diverse topics which have resulted in the successful publishing of this book. They have passed on their knowledge of decades through this book. To expedite this challenging task, the publisher supported the team at every step. A small team of assistant editors was also appointed to further simplify the editing procedure and attain best results for the readers.

Apart from the editorial board, the designing team has also invested a significant amount of their time in understanding the subject and creating the most relevant covers. They scrutinized every image to scout for the most suitable representation of the subject and create an appropriate cover for the book.

The publishing team has been an ardent support to the editorial, designing and production team. Their endless efforts to recruit the best for this project, has resulted in the accomplishment of this book. They are a veteran in the field of academics and their pool of knowledge is as vast as their experience in printing. Their expertise and guidance has proved useful at every step. Their uncompromising quality standards have made this book an exceptional effort. Their encouragement from time to time has been an inspiration for everyone.

The publisher and the editorial board hope that this book will prove to be a valuable piece of knowledge for researchers, students, practitioners and scholars across the globe.

List of Contributors

Keiko Hosohata, Ayaka Inada, Saki Oyama and Kazunori Iwanaga
Education and Research Center for Clinical Pharmacy, Osaka University of Pharmaceutical Sciences, Takatsuki, Osaka, Japan

Sang Soo Kim, Jong Ho Kim and Sang Heon Song
Department of Internal Medicine, Pusan National University School of Medicine, Yangsan, Gyeongsangnam-do, Republic of Korea
Biomedical Research Institute and Department of Internal Medicine, Pusan National University Hospital, Busan, Republic of Korea

Il Young Kim
Department of Internal Medicine, Pusan National University School of Medicine, Yangsan, Gyeongsangnam-do, Republic of Korea
Research Institute for Convergence of Biomedical Science and Technology and Department of Internal Medicine, Pusan National University Yangsan Hospital, Gyeongsangnam-do, Republic of Korea

Su Mi Lee
Division of Nephrology, Department of Internal Medicine, Dong-A University Hospital, Busan, Korea

Nika Kojc
Institute of Pathology, Faculty of Medicine, University of Ljubljana, Ljubljana, Slovenia

Eduardo Gomes Lima, Daniel Valente Batista, Eduardo Bello Martins and Whady Hueb
Department of Clinical Cardiology, Heart Institute (InCor), University of São Paulo, São Paulo, Brazil

Samuel N. Uwaezuoke and Ugo N. Chikani
College of Medicine, University of Nigeria/University of Nigeria Teaching Hospital, Enugu, Ituku-Ozalla, Nigeria
University of Nigeria Teaching Hospital, Enugu, Ituku-Ozalla, Nigeria

Ngozi R. Mbanefo
University of Nigeria Teaching Hospital, Enugu, Ituku-Ozalla, Nigeria

Ulrika Lundin
Sandoz GmbH, Kundl, Austria

Klaus M. Weinberger
Research Group for Clinical Bioinformatics, Institute for Electrical and Biomedical Engineering (IEBE), University for Health Sciences, Medical Informatics and Technology (UMIT), Hall in Tirol, Austria
sAnalytiCo Ltd, Belfast, United Kingdom
Weinberger and Weinberger Life Sciences Consulting, Lappersdorf, Germany

Marina Aksenova and Lev Shagam
Y.Veltischev Research and Clinical Institute for Pediatrics at the Pirogov Russian National Research Medical University, Moscow, Russia

Inès Jadot and Nathalie Caron
University of Namur, Namur, Belgium

Marilyn Duquesne, Anne-Emilie Declèves and Jean-Marie Colet
University of Mons, Mons, Belgium

Joëlle Nortier
Free University of Brussels, Brussels, Belgium

Index

www.ingramcontent.com/pod-product-compliance
Lightning Source LLC
Chambersburg PA
CBHW080300230326
41458CB00097B/5240